Question and Answers in PET/CT

Senthil Raja · Hian Liang Huang
Cindy Leung · Gopinath Gnanasegaran

Question and Answers in PET/CT

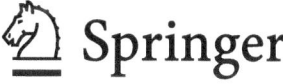 Springer

Senthil Raja
Department of Nuclear Medicine
and PET/CT
VPS Lakeshore Hospital
Kochi, Kerala, India

Cindy Leung
Department of Nuclear Medicine
Royal Free London NHS Foundation Trust
London, UK

Hian Liang Huang
Department of Nuclear Medicine
Singapore General Hospital
Bukit Merah, Central Region, Singapore

Gopinath Gnanasegaran
Department of Nuclear Medicine
Royal Free London NHS Foundation Trust
London, UK

ISBN 978-3-032-00820-6   ISBN 978-3-032-00821-3   (eBook)
https://doi.org/10.1007/978-3-032-00821-3

This Springer imprint is published by the registered company Springer Nature Switzerland AG
The registered company address is: Gewerbestrasse 11, 6330 Cham, Switzerland

If disposing of this product, please recycle the paper.

Preface

PET/CT imaging, a crucial tool for staging, restaging, assessing treatment response, and radiotherapy planning in various cancers, is extensively used in oncology and oncology clinical scenarios. It plays a significant role in multidisciplinary cancer meetings, contributing to effective patient management. This book is a valuable resource for professionals involved in these meetings.

Question and Answers in PET/CT is a book that caters to a wide range of professionals in the medical field. It is specifically aimed at referring clinicians, nuclear medicine physicians, radiologists, and physicians in training who regularly attend multidisciplinary meetings. However, it is also a valuable resource for Nuclear Medicine Technologists, Radiographers, and Nurses, ensuring that all members of the medical team can benefit from its comprehensive content.

We extend our heartfelt thanks to all the individuals who have contributed as authors to this book. Their expertise and dedication have been instrumental in creating this valuable resource. We would also like to express our gratitude to our family members, whose unwavering support has been a source of strength throughout this journey.

Kochi, Kerala, India   Senthil Raja

Singapore, Singapore   Hian Liang Huang

London, UK   Cindy Leung

London, UK   Gopinath Gnanasegaran

Contents

Contributors

Dr. Arun Visakh R Department of Nuclear Medicine, VPS Lakeshore Hospital, Kochi, Kerala, India

Dr. Arun Kumar Reddy Gorla Department of Nuclear Medicine, Sindhu Hospitals, Hyderabad, Telangana, India

Dr. Firuz Ibrahim Department of Nuclear Medicine, Burjeel Medical City, Abu Dhabi, UAE

Dr. Santhosh S Department of Nuclear Medicine, Dr. Rela Institute and Medical Centre, Chennai, Tamil Nadu, India

Basic Sciences

1. What does PET stand for?

   PET stands for positron emission tomography. A positron is the antiparticle of an electron. It is like the electron in terms of mass, except that, instead of a negative charge, it has a positive charge. Positrons are emitted by certain radioactive isotopes and undergo annihilation when interacting with a nearby electron, emitting two gamma rays of equal energy to the mass of the positron and electron, namely, 511 keV each. The isotopes tend to have excess protons compared to neutrons in their nuclei and emit positrons to increase nuclear stability. These are then detected by the scanner and transformed into a tomogram, a 3D representation of the body [1].

2. Why is PET paired with computed tomography (CT)?

   PET gives functional information regarding the intensity of tracer uptake in the cells of the studied lesion. While it provides location information, anatomical details usually need improvement. Pairing the PET with the CT offers a marriage of function and anatomy, allowing greater specificity in reading PET-CT. PET can sometimes be paired with magnetic resonance imaging (MRI), although technically more complex and expensive. The CT also provides attenuation correction by providing an attenuation map of the studied tissues. Previously, this was provided using external rotating radiation sources such as Germanium-68 [2]. However, this came at the cost of prolonged scanner time by approximately 40%. Of course, PET can be paired using software approaches with CT, as with MR. However, there are inherent advantages to using hardware pairing, such as ease of consistent patient positioning, little internal organ movement as scans are acquired close in time, and images are immediately available for concurrent review.

© The Author(s), under exclusive license to Springer Nature
Switzerland AG 2026
S. Raja et al., *Question and Answers in PET/CT*,
https://doi.org/10.1007/978-3-032-00821-3_1

3. What corrections must be made to the CT to pair it with PET?

The typical 70 keV photons of CT must be corrected to match the 511 keV photons of PET. They are then interpolated to the PET spatial resolution for attenuation correction map generation. Intravenous contrast use in CT generally does not pose problems with attenuation correction, as the change in CT attenuation minimally confounds the high-energy positrons. Modern scanners can usually distinguish between attenuation artifacts caused by dense material such as intravenous or oral contrast, metal, and catheters. However, reviewing the non-attenuation corrected images is sometimes revealing [3].

4. What are the options for the accompanying CT?

CT component of the PET/CT examination may be performed with low-dose settings and without intravenous contrast enhancement for attenuation correction and anatomical localization only. Alternatively, it can be performed as diagnostic-quality multislice CT with intravenous or oral contrast enhancement. The choice typically depends upon clinical need and department protocols, which remain a contention. If the low-dose protocol is selected, there is often recent prior or planned diagnostic contrast-enhanced imaging, although this is not always true.

5. What is the spatial resolution of PET?

Spatial resolution is an essential indicator of the scanner's performance. It can be measured using a point source and essentially represents the smallest distance between two points that the scanner can distinguish. Various factors, including the crystal size, positron range, acollinearity, decoding, penetration, and sampling error, limit this. Thus, the ultimate limit for PET-CT machines is thought to be 3 mm, although, in practice, it is difficult to achieve [4].

6. What are the crystals used in modern PET-CT machines?

The ideal scintillator crystal should have good stopping power for PET's high-energy 511 keV photons, which is usually achieved by using high atomic number elements with high densities. A fast, high-light output is also required for good energy and time resolution, allowing time-of-flight imaging and reducing image noise. Finally, a good light yield per photon is also sought [5]. Current scanners use either Lutetium oxy-orthosilicate ($Lu_2SiO_5(Ce)$, or LSO(Ce)), lutetium–yttrium oxy-orthosilicate ($Lu1.8Y0.2SiO_5(Ce)$, or LYSO(Ce), or Bismuth Germanate $Bi_4Ge_3O_{12}$, or BGO) crystals [6]. Recently, silicon photomultipliers have been developed, allowing for rapid, high-sensitivity digital imaging [7].

7. How low a concentration of tracer can be detected using nuclear medicine techniques?

Modern PET scanners have been shown to detect very low concentrations (in the region of 50 Bq/mL) of radiotracer in minimal concentrations of cells (104–105) in *in vitro* studies [8, 9]. The detectability of lesions *in vivo* may depend on the background tracer activity, adjacent physiological activity, and uptake time [10].

8. How does the PET scanner generate the images?

   The scanner detects photon pairs produced by the annihilation of positrons and electrons. These are then mapped onto lines of responses, which, when processed using iterative reconstruction methods, will localize the area where the annihilation event occurred and localize the tracer's position in the body. Modern scanners use CT or MRI to provide anatomical information about the locations of the annihilation events and can produce fused images with the PET data overlaid on anatomical CT or MR sequences [11]. Modern PET scanners typically use a ring of detectors to eliminate the need for rotating camera heads, and the latest iteration of PET scanners incorporates multiple rings of detectors in such a fashion to allow simultaneous whole-body imaging, albeit at a higher machine cost.

9. What are the corrections that the PET-CT scanner must make to the raw data to generate the images?

   (a) Scatter correction—in PET imaging, the phenomenon of photon scattering in the body's soft tissues can lead to inaccuracies in the scanner's line of flight. To address this, an energy window is placed around the expected 511 keV, effectively excluding photons with significantly lower energies due to Compton scatter, the primary cause of scatter in PET. This correction is crucial as it eliminates errors in the scanner's line of flight.

   (b) Random correction—coincidentally (or randomly), some photon pairs arrive from uncorrelated positron annihilations. Limiting the field of view and software correction can be reduced, but not eliminated.

   (c) Attenuation correction—as the photons interact with the body's soft tissues, they scatter, and the number of photons exiting the body decreases. If not corrected, photons from the body's surface will be very intense, and photons from areas with lower density, for example, the lungs, will be erroneously more intense than those adjacent to more dense areas, such as those inside the pelvis. Using either a rotating radioactive source or CT data, this can be corrected. However, suppose there are very dense structures in the field of view, such as metallic implants or dense barium. In that case, artifacts may be introduced into the corrected images, and knowledge of this potential pitfall is essential to accurate interpretation [12].

10. Is collimation required for PET imaging?

   In PET imaging, physical collimation is replaced by electronic collimation because the machine can detect coincidental photon emission (the emission of two photons from the positron annihilation event with a nearby electron) and thereby perform the corrections in question 7. This reduces the machine footprint, labor from changing collimators, and, most importantly, the technique's sensitivity [13].

   However, physical collimators can still be relied upon in certain special-use situations, such as small animal imaging, where high resolution is a priority over sensitivity. They can be used to correct for scatter and randoms, showcasing their physical adaptability. Yes, this may lead to a longer scanning time, but it is a trade-off that ensures we can meet the specific needs of our imaging tasks [14].

11. How does a cyclotron work?

Cyclotrons are commonly used to produce radioactive isotopes, which, in this case, are used in medical PET imaging. They accelerate and give energy to a proton (the nucleus of a hydrogen atom) and then cause a collision with a heavier target nucleus, creating a new isotope. The target nucleus depends on the positron emitter to be created. For example, 18F is produced by the bombardment of 18O, typically a commercially available stable isotope of oxygen [13].

Cyclotrons can cater to various needs with their versatile range of energies. Smaller cyclotrons, which produce medical isotopes like 18F, may only need to generate up to 15 MeV of energy. This is sufficient for the 10 MeV energy required to produce 18F-FDG, the most used PET tracer. On the other hand, larger and more expensive cyclotrons can accelerate protons with higher ranges of energy, showcasing the adaptability of this technology.

12. What are the radiation safety protection measures needed in PET imaging?

The requirement for an uptake phase, typically 60 min long, and the relatively higher energy of photons involved (511 keV, compared to the 140 keV of Technetium 99m) are challenges for radiation protection for staff engaged in PET imaging, and radiation doses tend to be higher than single-photon emission computed tomography (SPECT).

The first step in radiation safety protection in PET imaging is the design and layout of the PET center. The uptake rooms typically require lead or thick concrete shielding, and patients should be kept alone within them unless medically necessary. The flow of patients from the uptake rooms to the scanner should be as smooth and as short as possible to reduce exposure time. Procedure explanation, intravenous access, and glucose testing should all be done before radiotracer injection. Radiotracer injections should be performed via automated systems or, at the very least, incorporating heavy syringe shielding to reduce exposure. Structural shielding should be in place between the scanner room and the control room [15].

Tabletop shields and additional lead bricks strategically placed may further reduce staff exposure. Fortunately, because of the short half-lives of typical positron emitters being used, there is some mitigation for the high photon energy in terms of radiation protection.

Other radiation protection principles per radiology or SPECT scanning also apply, with the as low as reasonably achievable principle overriding. Exposure time should be reduced to a minimum, and distance should be observed.

References

1. Muehllehner G, Karp JS. Positron emission tomography. Phys Med Biol. 2006;51(13):R117.
2. Beyer T, Townsend DW, Brun T, Kinahan PE, Charron M, Roddy R, Jerin J, Young J, Byars L, Nutt R. A combined PET/CT scanner for clinical oncology. J Nucl Med. 2000;41(8):1369–79.
3. Townsend DW. Basic science of PET and PET/CT. In: Positron emission tomography. London: Springer; 2006. p. 1–16.

4. Moses WW. Fundamental limits of spatial resolution in PET. Nucl Instrum Methods Phys Res, Sect A. 2011;648:S236–40.
5. Nassalski A, Kapusta M, Batsch T, et al. Comparative study of scintillators for PET/CT detectors. IEEE Trans Nucl Sci. 2007;54(1):3–10. https://doi.org/10.1109/TNS.2006.890013.
6. Torres EI. PET/CT: underlying physics, instrumentation, and advances. Radiologia. 2017;59(5):431.
7. Surti S, Karp JS. Current status of PET technology. In: Advances in PET. Cham: Springer; 2020. p. 3–14.
8. Adler S, Seidel J, Choyke P, et al. Minimum lesion detectability as a measure of PET system performance. EJNMMI Phys. 2017;4(1):13. https://doi.org/10.1186/s40658-017-0179-2.
9. Sanchez-Crespo A, Jussing E, Björklund AC, et al. Hallmarks in prostate cancer imaging with Ga68-PSMA-11-PET/CT with reference to detection limits and quantitative properties. EJNMMI Res. 2018;8:27. https://doi.org/10.1186/s13550-018-0378-4.
10. Lechermann LM, Manavaki R, Attili B, et al. Detection limit of ^{89}Zr-labeled T cells for cellular tracking: an in vitro imagsing approach using clinical PET/CT and PET/MRI. EJNMMI Res. 2020;10:82. https://doi.org/10.1186/s13550-020-00667-5.
11. Moses WW. ConeBeam CT from image science to image guided surgery https://doi.org/10.1016/j.nima.2010.11.088.
12. Tong S, Alessio AM, Kinahan PE. Image reconstruction for PET/CT scanners: past achievements and future challenges. Imaging Med. 2010;2(5):529.
13. Daghighian F, Sumida R, Phelps ME. PET imaging: an overview and instrumentation. J Nucl Med Technol. 1990;18(1):5–13.
14. Walker M, Goorden M, Dinelle K, Ramakers R, Blinder S, Shirmohammad M, et al. Comparison of preclinical PET scanners: pinhole collimation vs. electronic collimation. J Nucl Med. 2014;55(supplement 1):1368.
15. Peet DJ, Morton R, Hussein M, Alsafi K, Spyrou N. Radiation protection in fixed PET/CT facilities – design and operation. Br J Radiol. 2012;85(1013):643–6. [cited 2020 Dec 28]

1. How does fluorine-18 fluorodeoxyglucose (18F-FDG) differ from glucose?

    18-Fluorodeoxyglucose is very similar to glucose, except that one of the hydroxyl groups is replaced by F18. F18 is produced by the bombardment of O18 in a cyclotron. [1]

2. How does 18F-FDG work in oncology?

    As a glucose analog, 18F-FDG enters cells primarily through glucose transport 1 (GLUT1) in the fasting state. GLUT1 is hyperexpressed in malignant cells compared to normal cells, the so-called Warburg effect [2]. Certain tumors also induce activated fibroblasts and inflammatory cells such as macrophages, which also contribute to the uptake of 18F-FDG. 18F-FDG is then phosphorylated by hexokinase II and then trapped in the cells as it cannot proceed further down the glycolysis pathway [3].

3. Why are some tumors 18F-FDG negative?

    Specific tumor subtypes are relatively less cellular than others. A good example would be a mucinous adenocarcinoma compared to an aggressive lymphoma. Thus, the signal from the 18F-FDG in a mucinous tumor may be lower due to interspersed mucinous material [4]. Other tumors may express low levels of GLUT1 and use the sodium-glucose cotransporters (SGLT) pathway. Some tumors may express low hexokinase and high glucose-6-phosphate, which dephosphorylates 18F-FDG-6-phosphate back to 18F-FDG and diffuses it out of the cells. The tumor microenvironment also plays a role—in general, a more hypoxic, poorly differentiated tumor will have more aggressive GLUT1 hyperexpression and vice versa [5]. P-glycoprotein is a drug efflux pump that is overexpressed in some lung cancers and cholangiocarcinomas, which may pump 18F-FDG out of the tumor cells [6].

© The Author(s), under exclusive license to Springer Nature
Switzerland AG 2026
S. Raja et al., *Question and Answers in PET/CT*,
https://doi.org/10.1007/978-3-032-00821-3_2

4. What are the mechanisms of uptake in common positron emission tomography (PET) tracers?

   The radiopharmaceutical uptake mechanism depends upon the organ or disease process being studied.

   (a) The GLUT1 transporter and the cellular microenvironment determine 18F-FDG uptake.
   (b) Other uptake mechanisms may include receptor site binding, as used in gallium-68 somatostatin receptor PET imaging and Prostate-Specific Membrane Antigen (PSMA) receptor PET imaging.
   (c) The normally operating metabolic cycles, such as for DNA synthesis or protein synthesis, can be used for imaging, and tracers such as 18F-fluorocholine and 18F-fluoroethyltyrosine, respectively, can be used to image these processes.
   (d) Radiopharmaceuticals may also be transcribed after partial metabolism. For example, 18F-MISO is metabolized by hypoxic cells and trapped, allowing imaging [7].

5. What are the methods of production of common PET tracers?

   18F-FDG can be synthesized by electrophilic or nucleophilic fluorination reaction. Nucleophilic fluorination is more popular because of its higher yield and shorter synthesis time. However, catalysts like kryptofix or tetrabutylammonium salts are required for 18F-FDG synthesis [8].

   Gallium-68—gallium-68 can be produced from a germanium-68/gallium-68 column generator, which is produced via a cyclotron [9]. Depending on the process being imaged, these are then chelated to various peptides or small molecules.

   Carbon-11, nitrogen-13, and oxygen-15—these short-lived PET emitters are generally all cyclotron-produced.

6. What are the quality control measures that need to be taken for PET radiopharmaceutials?

   The three major standards, Ph.Int., Ph. Eur., and USP, are available for 18F-FDG. These include physical parameters such as osmolality, pH, and appearance; radionuclide purity; radiochemical purity; and microbiological purity [10].

7. What is the normal biodistribution of 18F-FDG?

   Physiological biodistribution in humans depends upon GLUT1 expression.

   (a) The brain is an obligate user of glucose. Hence, there is intense activity under normal circumstances in the brain's gray matter.
   (b) Moderate uptake is seen in the liver, while under euglycemic conditions, mild uptake is seen in skeletal muscles, reflecting the storage metabolism of glucose under normal conditions.
   (c) Myocardial 18F-FDG uptake is variable as the myocardium can switch to using free fatty acids for metabolism under fasting conditions where a dearth of glucose is available.

(d) The kidneys, urine, and bladder reflect the clearance pathway for glucose and hence show variable, mainly intense tracer activity [11].

(e) The gut can also show variable uptake of 18F-FDG, and a few mechanisms are proposed due to intestinal permeability, gut microbiome, or even inflammation [12].

8. What affects the positron range of the tracers?

Positrons have different energies when emitted from the nuclei of the positron emitters, depending on the isotope being used—typical energies of emission range from 0.6 MeV for 18F to 3.4 MeV for 82Rb. The positrons then lose this energy in the surrounding tissues before annihilation to produce the photons detected by the PET scanner. The higher the energy of emission, the further the positron range, and therefore, this will lead to some loss of spatial resolution as a more extensive positron range represents a larger radius within which the true positron emission could have occurred.

9. What are the indications for commonly used PET tracers?

(a) 18F-FDG—oncology staging, restaging, response assessment and prognostication, neurology (dementia, tumors), cardiology (myocardial viability and inflammation), and infection/inflammation imaging

(b) 18F-NaF—positron-emitting radiopharmaceutical used for skeletal imaging

(c) 68Ga-PSMA/18F-PSMA—prostate cancer staging, biochemical recurrence, response assessment, and before PSMA therapy

(d) 68Ga-DOTA peptides—somatostatin receptor-positive tumor staging, restaging, response assessment, and before peptide receptor radionuclide therapy. While they image similar receptors, the affinity for the various subtypes differs, and scan findings may not be directly interchangeable.

(e) 13NH3, 82Rb—myocardial perfusion imaging

(f) 11C-acetate—imaging of hepatocellular carcinoma

(g) 18F-choline—imaging of prostate cancer, parathyroid adenoma

(h) 18F-MISO—hypoxia imaging

(i) 18F-DOPA—dopamine transporter imaging (in Parkinsonism, neuroendocrine tumors, and medullary thyroid carcinoma)

(j) 18F-FAPI, 68Ga-FAPI—oncological and non-oncological (cardiovascular, liver fibrosis/cirrhosis, arthritic disorders, IgG4 related disease, and pulmonary fibrosis/interstitial lung cases) [13]

10. What is the tracer principle?

The tracer principle is used in virtually all aspects of nuclear medicine. The concept is to have a small amount of radioactivity that is tagged to or "radiolabeled" to a peptide or other small molecule, which is then used to study biological and physiological processes, either with imaging with single-photon emission computed tomography or PET cameras or by quantification using radiation counters.

It has gained wide acceptance in the scientific community because of its high sensitivity of detection and high specificity in studying specific biological processes, in both pre-clinical and clinical work [14].

References

1. Ido T, Wan C, Casella J, et al. Labeled 2-deoxy-d-glucose analogs: 18F labeled 2-deoxy-2-fuoro-d-glucose, 2-deoxy-2- fuoro-d-mannose and 14C-2-deoxy-2-fuoro-d-glucose. J Label Compd Radiopharm. 1978;14:175–83.
2. Warburg OP, Negelein E. Uber den stofwechsel der carcinomzelle. Biochem Z. 1924;152:309–35.
3. Larson SM. 18 F-FDG imaging: molecular or functional? J Nucl Med. 2006;47:31N–2N.
4. Hofman MS, Hicks RJ. How we read oncologic FDG PET/CT. Cancer Imaging. 2016;16:35. https://doi.org/10.1186/s40644-016-0091-3.
5. O'Neill H, Malik V, Johnston C, Reynolds JV, O'Sullivan J. Can the efficacy of [18F]FDG-PET/CT in clinical oncology be enhanced by screening biomolecular profiles? Pharmaceuticals (Basel, Switzerland). 2019;12(1) https://doi.org/10.3390/ph12010016.
6. Smith TA. Influence of chemoresistance and p53 status on fluoro-2-deoxy-D-glucose incorporation in cancer. Nucl Med Biol. 2010;37(1):51–5. https://doi.org/10.1016/j.nucmedbio.2009.08.007. Epub 2009 Oct 3
7. Croteau E, Renaud JM, Richard MA, Ruddy TD, Bénard F, de Kemp RA. PET metabolic biomarkers for cancer. Biomark Cancer. 2016;8(suppl 2):BIC.S27483. [cited 2020 Nov 16] Available from: https://journals.sagepub.com/doi/full/10.4137/BIC.S27483
8. Fowler JS, Ido T. Initial and subsequent approach for the synthesis of 18FDG. Semin Nucl Med. 2002;32(1):6–12. https://doi.org/10.1053/snuc.2002.29270.
9. Oware W, Solanki KK, Bird N, Solanki C. Quality and validation of silica-based resin column of $^{68}Ge/^{68}Ga$ generator for use in medicinal product. World J Nucl Med. 2011;10:26–59.
10. Shukla J, Vatsa R, Garg N, Bhusari P, Watts A, Mittal BR. Quality control of positron emission tomography radiopharmaceuticals: an institutional experience. Indian J Nucl Med. 2013;28(4):200–6. https://doi.org/10.4103/0972-3919.121963.
11. Surasi DS, Bhambhvani P, Baldwin JA, Almodovar SE, O'Malley JP. 18F-FDG PET and PET/CT patient preparation: a review of the literature. J Nucl Med Technol. 2014;42(1):5–13.
12. Kang JY, Kim HN, Chang Y, et al. Gut microbiota and physiologic bowel ^{18}F-FDG uptake. EJNMMI Res. 2017;7(1):72. https://doi.org/10.1186/s13550-017-0318-8. Published 2017 Aug 31.
13. Chandekar KR, Prashanth A, Vinjamuri S, Kumar R. FAPI PET/CT imaging-an updated review. Diagnostics (Basel). 2023;13(12):2018.
14. Schwaiger M, Wester HJ, et al. J Nucl Med (Society of Nuclear Medicine). 2011;52:36S–41S. [cited 2020 Dec 28]

Patient Preparation

1. What information is needed before performing a positron emission tomography (PET)/ computed tomography (CT) scan?
   (a) Indication for the study
   (b) Patient's height and weight—this is used for calculations of standardized uptake value (SUV)
   (c) Blood sugar level
   (d) Presence of renal impairment, allergies (particularly to intravenous contrast agents), claustrophobia
   (e) Recently used medications, such as metformin, may impact biodistribution in fluorodeoxyglucose (FDG) studies
   (f) Pregnancy and breastfeeding status
   (g) Strenuous activity should be avoided for at least 12 h prior to the examination, or if done, the type of activity may be noted to increase reader confidence in the pattern of expected uptake.

2. Why do patients need to fast prior to FDG injection?
   Since FDG and glucose compete for the same transporters and hexokinase, the hyperglycemia caused by the post-prandial state may significantly modify the value of the semi-quantitative variables commonly used for estimating the uptake of FDG, including the SUV [1]. Parenteral nutrition and intravenous fluids containing glucose should be stopped at least 4 h before the injection of FDG. Plain water is allowed, but other beverages should be discouraged as trace amounts of sugar may be contained within. This restriction does not apply to many of the other PET tracers, where the mechanism of uptake and localization is unrelated to glucose metabolism.

S. Raja et al., *Question and Answers in PET/CT*, https://doi.org/10.1007/978-3-032-00821-3_3

3. What happens if there is uncontrolled hyperglycemia during FDG injection?

It is important to note that it is not hyperglycemia per se that renders the SUV inaccurate, but rather a state of hyperinsulinism, whether this is endogenous or exogenous. The presence of high levels of insulin results in increased uptake of FDG into skeletal muscles, myocardium, and the liver. This may result in poor target-to-background ratios in the tumors and falsely low SUV values due to the redistribution of FDG [2].

4. How to deal with hyperglycemia prior to FDG PET/CT?

In oncological studies, in general, it is recommended for the blood glucose level < 11.1 11.1 recommended for the generalto the redistribution of FDG [2]. in the tumoism, whether this is endogenous or exogenous. The presence of high levels of insulin results in increased ue recommended levels are between 7 and 8.3 mmol/L (126 and 150 mg/dL). However, in clinical practice, there is often pressure to conserve expensive tracer and scanner time, not to mention inconvenience to patients. There are various methods to manage hyperglycemia, including prolonged fasting, delayed injection of FDG, intravenous hydration, and intravenous insulin [3].

5. Why is there a waiting time between tracer injection and scanning?

A delay between the injection and the imaging time, the so-called uptake time, is used in many indications for FDG PET, including oncological, infection, cardiovascular, and neurological imaging. The recommended delay is 60 min, with an acceptable range of 55–75 min, but, in practice, there may be longer waiting times due to logistical issues. It is important to note such differences when comparing scans, especially in the context of clinical trials. Many other PET tracers also incorporate an uptake time, including gallium-68 Prostate-Specific Membrane Antigen (PSMA) and tetraazacyclododecanetetraacetic acid (DOTA) peptides. The purpose is to allow enough time for the tracer to be circulated through the body and cleared from the blood pool into the tissues of interest, and finally to bind to the target lesions of interest, with clearance of the background activity to allow for a good target-to-background ratio of uptake and so increase conspicuity [4]. Newer scanners will enable the study of the kinetics of this process; however, most applications are currently in research [5].

6. Why are patients requested to drink fluids and void before scanning?

Adequate hydration is essential to ensure a sufficiently low concentration of FDG in the urine (fewer artifacts) and for radiation safety reasons. For example, 1 L of water is suggested during the 2 h before injection. Where necessary, account for the volume of water in the oral contrast agent if it is to be given for a diagnostic CT scan. Voiding before the scan also helps to reduce artifacts from intense excreted urinary FDG activity, which may obscure lesions in the pelvis [6].

7. What is the "cardiac sarcoid diet" preparation and what is it for?

The myocardium preferentially uses glucose as a substrate for metabolism. This leads to physiologically intense FDG uptake in normal circumstances. However, during periods of fasting, the myocardium can "switch" to using free fatty acids for metabolism [7]. In some instances, it is beneficial, if not essential, to suppress the physiological uptake of FDG to assess for the presence of infection (in the case of suspected cardiac device infection or endocarditis) and inflammation (in the case of sarcoidosis) or even malignancy in the heart.

Options available to suppress myocardial uptake include:

(a) High-fat-enriched diet lacking carbohydrates for 12–24 h before the scan
(b) Prolonged fasting period of 12–18 h before injection of FDG. The easiest to tolerate may involve having dinner at 6 pm and performing the scan at noon the next day, with missing breakfast and having a late lunch.
(c) Intravenous heparin of 50 IU/kg approximately 15 min before FDG injection [8]

8. What are the contraindications for PET/CT scanning?

There are no absolute contraindications for a PET scan. However, the study may not be suitable for pregnant women. Performing PET/CT in pregnancy should be avoided as much as possible. The benefit versus risk should be discussed with the nuclear medicine specialist. If scanning is performed, the most significant source of radiation exposure to the fetus would be from the excreted activity in the urinary bladder, hence the importance of voiding before scanning. Dosimetry calculations to estimate the fetal dose should then be calculated, and the case should be referred to the institutional radiation safety officer for evaluation.

Breastfeeding patients can undergo PET/CT. Depending on the tracer, there may be excretion into the breast milk, although the half-lives of current commonly used PET radiopharmaceuticals tend to be short-lived. The current expression of breast milk may need to be discarded or stored for multiple half-lives, but, in general, there is no need to cease breastfeeding for PET imaging.

Poorly controlled diabetes should not represent an absolute contraindication, as the study can still be read, although diagnostic sensitivity and comparison accuracy will be reduced.

In patients with renal impairment or contrast allergy, the use of accompanying intravenous CT contrast agents has to be cautious. In many cases, the same information can be obtained with a non-contrast CT for anatomical correlation.

Large patients weighing more than 90 kg should not be a contraindication to PET/CT, although the acquisition time will be longer due to the attenuation by body tissues. There are weight limits to the scanning tables, which are vendor and scanner-dependent [9].

9. What are the field of view options for PET/CT scanning?

This depends upon the indication for the study and may sometimes vary between institutions. Local department protocols should be adhered to.

Whole body from this depends upon the indication for the study and may sometimes vary between institutions. Local department protocols should be adhered to.

(a) Whole body from the skull vertex through the feet

This option is commonly used for pediatric patients, pyrexia of unknown origin, cardiac infection (for septic emboli), and malignancies which may involve the distal lower limbs more commonly, such as melanoma, myeloma, sarcomas, and T-cell lymphomas. However, this option increases the imaging time of the scans.

(b) Skull base or vertex to mid-thighs

Imaging from the vertex to the mid-thighs is the most used option for FDG PET/CT imaging of malignancy. Whether to include the brain or start from the skull base is controversial, given the variable detection frequency of brain metastases with the high physiological background gray matter FDG activity, and local department protocols should be considered. Arms along the sides may produce artifacts over the torso. For optimal body imaging, the arms should be elevated over the head if tolerated by the patient. The arms should be positioned along the sides for optimal imaging of the head and neck.

(c) Limited region (e.g., brain only or chest only)

This option usually allows for a longer PET acquisition time of specific regions of interest, for example, the brain for dementia or intracerebral malignancy viability, and the chest for cases of suspected myocardial inflammation [10].

(d) This option is commonly used for pediatric patients, pyrexia of unknown origin, cardiac infection (for septic emboli), and malignancies which may involve the distal lower limbs more commonly, such as melanoma, myeloma, sarcomas, and T-cell lymphomas. However, this option increases the imaging time of the scans.

(e) Skull base or vertex to mid-thighs

This option is the most commonly used for FDG PET/CT imaging of malignancy. Whether to include the brain or start from the skull base is a matter of controversy given the variable detection frequency of brain metastases with the high physiological background gray matter FDG activity, and local department protocols should be considered. Arms along the sides may produce artifacts over the torso. For optimal imaging of the body, the arms should be elevated over the head if tolerated by the patient. For optimal imaging of the head and neck, the arms should be positioned along the sides.

(f) Limited region (e.g., brain only or chest only)

This option usually allows for a longer PET acquisition time of specific regions of interest, for example, the brain for dementia or intracerebral malignancy viability, and the chest for cases of suspected myocardial inflammation [10].

10. How should the uptake time be spent?

Patients should be seated or recumbent in a quiet room to reduce muscle uptake, which may obscure lesions. In cold climates, heated blankets and a relatively warm waiting room may decrease brown fat activity, which helps interpret the neck. Patients may sleep if the brain is not explicitly being evaluated, such as in cases of suspected dementia; otherwise, they should have their eyes open but not reading, as this will activate the intraocular muscles. For cases of suspected dementia, the occipital lobe activity needs to be assessed; hence, sleeping or having eyes closed during the uptake phase may confound interpretation [11].

References

1. Tenley N, Corn DJ, Yuan L, Lee Z. The effect of fasting on PET imaging of hepatocellular carcinoma. J Cancer Ther. 2013;4(2):561–7. https://doi.org/10.4236/jct.2013.42071.
2. Evangelista L, Gori S, Rubini G, et al. Management of hyperglycemia in oncological patients scheduled for an FDG-PET/CT examination. Clin Translat Imaging. 2019;7:447–50. https://doi.org/10.1007/s40336-019-00347-y.
3. Pattison DA, MacFarlane LL, Callahan J, Kane EL, Akhurst T, Hicks RJ. Personalised insulin calculator enables safe and effective correction of hyperglycaemia prior to FDG PET/CT. EJNMMI Res. 2019;9(1):15. https://doi.org/10.1186/s13550-019-0480-2. Published 2019 Feb 8.
4. Wangerin KA, Muzi M, Peterson LM, et al. Effect of ^{18}F-FDG uptake time on lesion detectability in PET imaging of early stage breast cancer [published correction appears in Tomography; 2(3):238]. Tomography. 2015;1(1):53–60. https://doi.org/10.18383/j.tom.2015.00151.
5. Huang J, O'Sullivan F. An analysis of whole body tracer kinetics in dynamic PET studies with application to image-based blood input function extraction. IEEE Trans Med Imaging. 2014;33(5):1093–108. https://doi.org/10.1109/TMI.2014.2305113.
6. Boellaard R, Delgado-Bolton R, Oyen WJ, Giammarile F, Tatsch K, Eschner W, Verzijlbergen FJ, Barrington SF, Pike LC, Weber WA, Stroobants S. FDG PET/CT: EANM procedure guidelines for tumour imaging: version 2.0. Eur J Nucl Med Mol Imaging. 2015;42(2):328–54.
7. Erba PA, Lancellotti P, Vilacosta I, Gaemperli O, Rouzet F, Hacker M, et al. Recommendations on nuclear and multimodality imaging in IE and CIED infections. Eur J Nucl Med Mol Imaging. 2018;45(10):1795–815.
8. College of Radiology A. ACR-SPR practice parameter for performing FDG-PET/CT.
9. Delbeke D, Coleman RE, Guiberteau MJ, Brown ML, Royal HD, Siegel BA, et al. Combined Procedure Guidelines of SNM, EANM and BNMS for SPECT/CT and PETCT. Imaging. 2011:1–16.
10. Boellaard R, Delgado-Bolton R, Oyen WJG, Giammarile F, Tatsch K, Eschner W, et al. FDG PET/CT: EANM procedure guidelines for tumour imaging: version 2.0. Eur J Nucl Med Mol Imaging. 2015;42:328–54. https://doi.org/10.1007/s00259-014-2961-x.
11. Waxman AD, Herholz K, Lewis DH, Herscovitch P, Minoshima S, Ichise M, et al. Society of nuclear medicine procedure guideline for FDG PET brain imaging.

Brain

4

1. What are the common positron emission tomography (PET) tracers used in brain imaging?

    Commonly used PET tracers for brain imaging are

    A. Glucose analog—^{18}F-fluorodeoxyglucose (^{18}F-FDG)
    B. Radiolabeled amino acids—^{11}C-methionine , ^{18}F-fluoroethyl tyrosine, and ^{18}F fluoro dihydroxyphenylalanine
    C. Nucleoside analog ^{18}F-fluorothymidine

    Other PET tracers that may play a role in the evaluation of brain tumors are as follows:

    A. Hypoxia sensitive agents—^{18}F-fluoromisonidazole
    B. ^{11}C-acetate
    C. ^{11}C-choline
    D. Somatostatin analogs (e.g., ^{68}Ga-DOTATOC and ^{68}Ga-DOTATATE) [1]

2. What is the role of ^{18}F-FDG in dementia?

    Neurodegenerative dementias are associated with specific patterns of regional hypometabolism. FDG PET is useful in the early diagnosis of Alzheimer's dementia (AD) with minimal cognitive impairment patients. It may also help differentiate various dementias such as AD, dementia with Lewy bodies (DLB), and frontotemporal dementia (FTD) if classic patterns of hypometabolism are present. It is also helpful in differentiating pseudodementia from true dementia [2].

    Further evaluation with more specific tracers, such as amyloid or tau PET or I-123 ioflupane, may be required to elucidate the etiology of dementia further.

3. What is the role of ^{18}F-FDG in neuro-oncology?

Primary indications for 18F-FDG in current clinical neuro-oncology are as follows:

- Differentiating recurrent high-grade glioma or brain metastases from radiation necrosis
- Distinguishing CNS lymphoma from infectious processes (e.g., Toxoplasmosis) in the brain, particularly in immunocompromised patients [3].

4. What is the role of 18F-FDG in epilepsy?

FDG PET may help lateralize or localize the epileptogenic focus in the following situations:

A. Focal epilepsy with normal magnetic resonance imaging (MRI)
B. Imaging is discordant with electrophysiology
C. Bilateral or multiple lesions on MRI
   It is also helpful in guiding intracranial electrode placement [2].

5. What is the role of 18F-FDG in movement disorders?

18F-FDG PET can be helpful to distinguish among patient groups with extrapyramidal neurodegenerative movement disorders such as Parkinson's disease (PD), progressive supranuclear palsy (PSP), multiple system atrophy (MSA), and corticobasal degeneration (CBD) as well as other movement disorders such as essential tremors, ataxia, and dystonia [4].

6. What are the common patient preparations for 18F-FDG Brain imaging?

Fasting for at least 4 h before tracer injection.

Avoid caffeine, alcohol, or drugs that may affect cerebral glucose metabolism.

Check blood glucose level (ideally not greater than 150–200 mg/dL).

Environmental conditions: resting state, patient with eyes open and ears unoccluded in a quiet, dimly lit room, with minimal background noise.

Start intravenous line for 18F-FDG administration at least 10 min before tracer injection to avoid activation of pain centers.

In the preoperative evaluation of epilepsy, monitoring should ideally start 2 h before injection to ensure that FDG is not administered in an ictal state, confounding interpretation [5].

7. What is the normal variability of regional FDG uptake?

The brain shows intense physiological 18F-FDG uptake, with higher activity in the gray matter than the white matter (normal gray/white matter activity ratio ranges from 2.5 to 4.1).

18F-FDG uptake is usually higher in the frontal, parietal, and occipital areas than in the temporal cortex, and the basal ganglia have slightly higher activity than the cortex.

Moreover, focal areas of increased uptake were observed in normal subjects' frontal eye fields, posterior cingulate cortex, and visual cortex, particularly with visual activation during the uptake phase.

Metabolic activity is lower in the medial temporal cortex, including hippo-campal areas.

Slight asymmetries in 18F-FDG uptake have been observed in the Wernicke area, frontal eye fields, and angular gyri, generally less than 10% [6].

8. What is the role of FDG PET quantitation in brain tumors?

Common quantitative parameters used in brain tumors are Standard uptake values (SUV) and Activity ratios (equivalent to SUV ratios). Whilst it is sug-gested that these can differentiate radiation injury from a viable brain tumor, and suggest aggressiveness in grade and behavior, this is a controversial area, and fixed cut-offs have gradually fallen out of favor.

Quantitation and thresholding could be used to delineate the gross tumor volume for radiotherapy planning [1, 7]. Quantitation and thresholding could be used to delineate the gross tumor volume for radiotherapy planning [1, 7].

9. What is the relationship between FDG uptake and brain tumor grade?

FDG uptake is usually directly proportional to the grade of brain tumor; however, there are exceptions, and histological correlation is paramount.

Ratios of 18F-FDG uptake in tumors to that in white matter (ratio of tumor to white matter 1.5) or gray matter (ratio of tumor to gray matter 0.6) were able to identify and distinguish benign brain tumors (grades I and II) from malignant brain tumors (grades III and IV) in some studies [8, 9].

10. What are the advantages of 18F-FDG-PET in brain tumors?

The uptake of 18F-FDG by brain tumors is not flow-dependent.

The 18F-FDG uptake by gliomas correlates with tumor grade and prognosis.

FDG also usually has greater uptake in recurrent high-grade gliomas than in radiation necrosis, which may be used to distinguish recurrent tumors from the effects of radiation therapy.

It may be helpful in differentiating CNS lymphoma from opportunistic infections in immunocompromised patients [3].

11. What are the limitations of 18F-FDG-PET in brain tumors?

High and regionally variable FDG uptake in normal brains often makes delineating brain tumors difficult.

FDG is a non-specific tracer. Inflammatory lesions, including brain abscesses, granulomatous inflammation for both infectious and noninfectious causes, and normal brain parenchyma adjacent to subacute intraparenchymal hemorrhages, can also have a high uptake of 18F-FDG, decreasing the specificity of 18F-FDG in differentiating tumor from non-malignant etiology [1].

12. What are the typical of 18F-FDG findings in dementia?

AD—temporoparietal hypometabolism is a characteristic finding that includes the precuneus and the posterior cingulate cortex in the early disease course. In advanced cases, hypometabolism is also seen in the frontal lobes— sparing of the primary somatosensory cortex, visual cortex, the basal ganglia and thalami, and the cerebellum. This pattern of hypometabolism may be asym-metric but is usually bilateral.

DLB—is characterized by a posterior predominant, occipitoparietal hypometabolism involving the primary visual and occipital association areas with relatively preserved metabolism in medial temporal and posterior cingulate cortices, distinguishing DLB from AD.

FTD—behavioral or frontal variant predominately frontal hypometabolism, with varying involvement of the anterior cingulate cortex and anterior temporal lobes.

Semantic dementia—is associated with predominantly anterior temporal lobe hypometabolism that is usually asymmetric.

Progressive nonfluent aphasia—even more asymmetric, associated with left perisylvian hypometabolism.

Vascular dementia—asymmetric hypometabolism and often involves brain regions spared in Alzheimer's and other neurodegenerative dementias, including primary somatosensory cortex and subcortical structures such as the basal ganglia and thalami.

Pseudodementia—normal [2].

13. What are the typical 18F-FDG findings in neuro-oncology?

In low-grade brain tumors, FDG uptake is considerably lower, mostly similar to that in normal white matter.

In high-grade brain tumors, FDG uptake is usually more than white matter uptake and may be lower than or similar to that of normal gray matter.

A few very high-grade tumors, such as glioblastoma mutiforme or CNS lymphoma, might show higher uptake than the physiological gray matter uptake [10].

14. What are the typical of 18F-FDG findings in epilepsy?

Focal hypometabolism on interictal FDG-PET is the typical finding seen in epilepsy. The hypometabolic area elicited on FDG PET is known as the functional deficit zone, which is usually much larger than the epileptogenic zone as PET findings reflect the neuronal activity not only at the site of ictal onset but also in areas of ictal spread and postictal depression [11].

15. What are the typical of 18F-FDG findings in movement disorders?

PD—FDG hypermetabolism in the striatum in early presentation (before use of DA replacement therapy/with therapy withdrawal). Hypometabolism occurs in the parietal association cortex and the occipital cortex in advanced cases.

MSA—Parkinson type has symmetric FDG hypometabolism in the putamen.

MSA—cerebellar type has prominent hypometabolism in the pons and cerebellum.

PSP—symmetric FDG hypometabolism in the striatum (differentially involving the caudate nuclei) and in the frontal lobe neocortices, particularly dorsal prefrontal and mesial frontal aspects.

CBD—asymmetric hypometabolism in the precentral and postcentral gyri, the striatum, and the thalamus

Huntington's disease—hypometabolism in the striatum and mild hypometabolism in the frontal and temporal cortex [12, 13].

References

1. Sharma A, McConathy J. Overview of PET tracers for brain tumor imaging. PET Clin. 2013;8:129–46.
2. Nasrallah I, Dubroff J. An overview of PET neuroimaging. Semin Nucl Med. 2013;43:449–61.
3. Herholz K, Langen KJ, Schiepers C, Mountz JM. Brain tumors. Semin Nucl Med. 2012;42:356–70.
4. Berti V, Pupi A, Mosconi L, et al. PET/CT in diagnosis of movement disorders. Ann N Y Acad Sci. 2011;1228:93–108.
5. Varrone A, Asenbaum S, Vander Borght T, et al. EANM procedure guidelines for PET brain imaging using [18F]FDG, version 2. Eur J Nucl Med Mol Imaging. 2009;36:2103–10.
6. Berti V, Mosconi L, Pupi A. Brain: normal variations and benign findings in fluorodeoxyglucose-PET/computed tomographyimaging. PET Clin. 2014;9:129–40.
7. Senthamizhchelvan S, Zaidi H. Novel quantitative techniques in hybrid (PET-MR) imaging of brain tumors. PET Clin. 2013;8(2):219–32.
8. Delbeke D, Meyerowitz C, Lapidus RL, et al. Optimal cutoff levels of F-18 fluorodeoxyglucose uptake in the differentiation of low-grade from high-grade brain tumors with PET. Radiology. 1995;195:47–52.
9. Song PJ, Lu QY, Li MY, Li X, Shen F. Comparison of effects of 18F-FDG PET-CTand MRI in identifying and grading gliomas. J Biol Regul Homeost Agents. 2016;30:833–8.
10. Chen W. Clinical applications of PET in brain tumors. J Nucl Med. 2007;48:1468–81.
11. Tamber MS, Mountz JM. Advances in the diagnosis and treatment of epilepsy. Semin Nucl Med. 2012;42:371–86.
12. Frey KA. Molecular imaging of extrapyramidal movement disorders. Semin Nucl Med. 2017;47:18–30.
13. Roussakis AA, Piccini P. PET imaging in Huntington's disease. J Huntington's Dis. 2015;4:287–96.

Lung Cancer

5

1. What are the common histological subtypes of primary lung cancer?
   - (a) Squamous cell carcinoma
   - (b) Adenocarcinoma
   - (c) Small/oat cell carcinoma
   - (d) Large cell carcinoma [1]

2. What is the role of ^{18}F-fluorodeoxyglucose (18F-FDG) positron emission tomography (PET)-computed tomography (CT) in lung cancer?

   The role of 18F-FDG PET in lung cancer includes the following:
   - (a) Malignancy risk assessment of solitary pulmonary nodule (SPN)
   - (b) Initial staging (1. Staging of patients considered for radical treatment of non-small cell lung cancer NSCLC. 2. Staging of patients with small-cell lung cancer with limited disease on CT being considered for radical therapy)
   - (c) Re-staging after induction therapy
   - (d) Radiotherapy planning
   - (e) Finding the appropriate site of biopsy [2]

3. What is the complete description that characterizes a solitary pulmonary nodule?
   - (a) Single, round, well-circumscribed lung opacity
   - (b) Size ≤ 3 cm in diameter
   - (c) Completely surrounded by pulmonary parenchyma
   - (d) Not associated with atelectasis, lymph node enlargement, pneumonia, and pleural effusion [3]

With Contributions by Dr. Santhosh S

4. What is true regarding the incidence of SPN?
    (a) 0.09–0.2% of all chest X-ray (CXR) scans will incidentally detect pulmo-
        nary nodules.
    (b) 31% of patients undergoing cardiac CT scans for coronary calcium scoring
        have incidental findings of pulmonary nodules (in specific populations).
    (c) In lung cancer screening trials, 7% of CXR scans obtained from previously
        healthy individuals contain pulmonary nodules.
    (d) CT scans to screen for lung cancer detect nodules in 8–51% of individuals
        screened [4, 5].

5. What is true regarding the role of 18F-FDG PET in diagnosing lung cancer?
    (a) In regions with endemic infectious diseases, the specificity of FDG-PET
        for lung cancer diagnosis is lower (61%) than in non-endemic regions
        (77%) [6, 7].
    (b) Sensitivity does not change appreciably depending on the status of the
        endemic infection.
    (c) FDG-PET is discouraged in patients with a high pre-test probability of
        malignancy (>60%) or in nodules that measure <10 mm, although this may
        be used for staging purposes [8].

6. What is the role of 18F-FDG PET in re-staging lung cancer?
    (a) Exclude disease progression
    (b) Exclude interval development of metastatic disease [2]

7. What is the role of 18F-FDG PET in the assessment of treatment response in
   lung cancer?
    (a) Metabolic criteria using PET/CT could accurately predict response and dis-
        ease progression early in targeted therapy, compared to morphologic crite-
        ria on CT scans.
    (b) 18F-FDG-PET/CT after one treatment cycle is predictive of the outcome
        of first-line chemotherapy with bevacizumab in patients with advanced
        non-squamous NSCLC.
    (c) In locally advanced NSCLC, 18F-FDG metabolic response assessed after
        only two cycles of IC-LDRT predicts the prognosis [9–11].

8. What is true regarding 18F-FDG in various lung cancers?
    (a) Adenocarcinoma *in situ* has a significantly low SUV compared to most
        other subtypes [12]
    (b) SUVmax of BAC < adeno < adenosquamous < squamous < large cell
        carcinoma
    (c) SUVmax of pathological grade III > II > I carcinoma [13]

9. What are the pooled sensitivity, specificity, positive likelihood ratio (PLR),
   negative likelihood ratio (NLR) of 18F-FDG in assessment of mediastinal nodal
   disease in lung cancer?
    (a) 0.65, 0.93, 8.46, and 0.38 [14]

10. What are the sensitivity, specificity, positive predictive value (PPV), and negative predictive value (NPV) of 18F-FDG in the assessment of distant metastasis?
    (a) 72%, 100%, 97%, and low NPV for brain metastasis [15]
    (b) 94.3%, 98.8%, 90%, and 99.3% for skeletal metastasis [16]
    (c) 97%, 91%, 11.1 PLR, and 0.04 NLR for adrenal metastasis [17]

11. What are the criteria for PET positivity in indeterminate pulmonary nodules?
    (a) FDG-avidity in >8 mm solid non-calcified or part-solid nodule is suspicious for malignancy.
    (b) SUV greater than the baseline mediastinal blood pool is a criterion for positive PET [2].

12. What are the pooled sensitivity, specificity, PLR, and NLR in SPN?
    (a) 91.7%, 82.3%, 5.18, and 0.10 [18]

13. What is the role of 18F-FDG PET-CT in T staging?
    (a) Better determination of chest wall infiltration (potentially resectable T3a)
    (b) Better determination of mediastinal invasion
    (c) Differentiate tumor from peritumoral atelectasis [19]

14. What is the role of 18F-FDG PET-CT in N staging?
    (a) To allow direct surgical resection in tumors ≤ 3 cm in the outer third of the lung with negative PET
    (b) To direct biopsy, either endobronchial ultrasound (EBUS)-guided or mediastinoscopic [20]

15. What is the role of 18F-FDG PET-CT in M staging?
    (a) Not an ideal tool for the evaluation of brain metastasis
    (b) Is useful for all clinical stages for evaluation of unsuspected distant metastasis
    (c) Prevents futile thoracotomies [21]

16. What are the common pitfalls of 18F-FDG PET-CT in staging lung cancer?
    (a) Iatrogenic microembolism could lead to focal intrapulmonary FDG uptake [22]
    (b) High FDG uptake in normal brain parenchyma precludes evaluation of brain metastasis [23]
    (c) False-positive uptakes in infection, inflammation, and infarction [24]
    (d) False-negative 18F-FDG PET-CT findings due to misregistration, fewer FDG-avid histological subtypes, and small (<8 mm) lesions [5, 25, 26]

17. What are the advantages and limitations of 18F-FDG PET-CT in the assessment of mediastinal lymph node status?
    (a) PET-CT can miss occult nodal metastasis in T2 disease and all centrally located tumors regardless of size.
    (b) Sensitivity of nodal disease is better for squamous compared to adenocarcinoma.
    (c) When N1 nodal involvement is suspected, preoperative mediastinal staging is indicated irrespective of the PET-negative status of N2 nodes [2, 20, 27].

18. What types of lung mass or nodule location are assessable for biopsy?
    (a) Bronchus sign on CT predicts a higher diagnostic yield from flexible bronchoscopy.
    (b) The diagnostic yield of bronchoscope-guided systems for sampling of peripheral lung nodules is 60.9% and 82.5% for lesions ≤2 cm and >2 cm, respectively.
    (c) Transthoracic needle biopsy (TTNB) is preferred for nodules located near the chest wall or for deeper lesions if fissures do not need to be traversed and there is no surrounding emphysema.
    (d) Bronchoscopic techniques are favored for nodules near a patent bronchus and in individuals at high risk for pneumothorax following TTNB [8, 28].

19. What are non-FDG tracers in imaging lung cancer?
    (a) 18F-Fluorothymidine (FLT) is a specific marker of cell proliferation
    (b) 18F-Fluoromisonidazole (F-MISO) is a marker for hypoxia and helpful in planning radiotherapy
    (c) 18F/11C-methionine is a marker of protein synthesis and may be employed for evaluating brain metastasis [29]

20. What is the role FDG PET-CT in guidance of invasive procedures?
    (a) Facilitates percutaneous biopsy of FDG-avid metastatic bone lesions in suspected advanced lung cancer [30].
    (b) Improves the accuracy of CT-guided FNA of lung lesions.
    (c) Decreases the rate of sampling error.
    (d) Improves targeting of mediastinal lymph nodes [31].

21. What is the role of 18F-FDG PET-CT in the management of non-small cell lung cancer?
    (a) By accurate staging, avoid futile thoracotomy [32].
    (b) Early 18F-FDG-PET assessment allows identification of NSCLC patients who do not benefit from first-line chemotherapy [33].
    (c) High values of SUVmax, metabolic tumor volume, and total lesion glycolysis predict a higher risk of recurrence or death in patients with surgical resection of NSCLC [34].

22. What is the role of 18F-FDG PET-CT in the management of small cell lung cancer?
    (a) To differentiate between limited and extensive disease during initial staging [35].

23. What is the role of respiratory gated 18F-FDG PET-CT scan in lung cancer patients?
    (a) Improves the sensitivity for lower lobe lesions and small lesions (< 15 mm) [36].
    (b) Allows a more accurate definition of the lesion volume and improves the quantitation of tracer activity [37].
    (c) Improves the accuracy of lymph node staging [38].

24. What is the best role of 18F-FDG PET-CT in radiotherapy planning in NSCLC?
    (a) To improve target delineation accuracy, especially when there is atelectasis or contraindications to intravenous CT contrast
    (b) Other potential roles include:
        • Imaging of lesions not apparent on CT or MRI, such as unsuspected lymph nodes or distant metastases
        • To facilitate dose painting/dose sculpting in intensity modulated radiotherapy
        • "Response-adapted therapy," where changes to target volumes could potentially be made during a treatment course [2, 39]

25. What are the normal variants and artifacts in 18F-FDG PET-CT in imaging thoracic malignancies?
    (a) Respiratory artifact resulting in liver metastasis misregistered to the lung mimicking lung metastasis.
    (b) Physiological FDG uptake in lipomatous hypertrophy of the interatrial septum can mimic metastasis.
    (c) FDG avidity in talc pleurodesis can mimic pleural metastasis [40]

26. What is the role of 18F-FDG PET-CT in imaging bronchial carcinoids?
    (a) Complementary role to DOTA-(Tyr3)-octreotate (DOTATATE) PET-CT
    (b) Can differentiate hamartomas from carcinoids
    (c) Atypical carcinoids tend to have increased but overlapping SUVmax when compared with typical carcinoids.
    (d) More sensitive for higher-grade tumors and positive FDG-PET associated with poor survival [41–43]

27. What is the role of 18F-FDG PET-CT in radiotherapy planning in small cell lung cancer?
    (a) In patients with limited disease, target volume definition is performed within 4 weeks before radiotherapy. It is also useful in accurate tumour and nodal delineation, reduces interobserver variability, refines treatment plans and can assess treatment response after radiotherapy [35].

28. What are the limitations of 18F-FDG PET-CT in radiotherapy planning?
    (a) Variations in the methodology of tumor target volume delineation
    (b) Blurring effect at the edges hampers the exact delineation of FDG-avid tissues
    (c) Low signal-to-background ratio [44, 45]

29. Explain about the cost effectiveness of 18F-FDG PET-CT for characterizing pulmonary nodules?
    (a) Cost-effectiveness of the different management strategies of the SPN depends on the malignancy pretest probability.
    (b) PET is not recommended as the initial test in almost all circumstances.

(c) FDG PET-CT is cost-effective at low to moderate pre-test probabilities (5–65%).

(d) PET is not recommended as the initial test only when the pretest probability is very high (>0.90%) [8, 46, 47].

30. What is the management of non-FDG avid lung nodules?
(a) At low clinical probability (<30–40%), follow-up CT should be done. Such serial CT scans should be performed at 3–6, 9–12, and 18–24 months, using thin sections and noncontrast, low-dose techniques.
(b) When the probability of malignancy is low to moderate (~10% to 60%), nonsurgical biopsy should be done [8].

31. What is true regarding the management of lung cancers?
(a) PET can be indicated with the aim of pre-treatment staging and not for characterizing the nodule in a patient with a high pre-test probability (>65%).
(b) Positive PET/CT scan findings for distant disease need pathologic or radiologic confirmation.
(c) If the PET/CT scan is positive for the mediastinum, the lymph node status needs pathologic confirmation [2, 8].

32. What are the advantages and limitations of FDG PET-CT in detecting adrenal metastasis?
(a) Calculating quantitative standardized uptake values is less useful for PET characterizing adrenal masses.
(b) Most adrenal masses can be characterized by using FDG PET, and subsequent imaging to characterize the adrenal lesions generally should be unnecessary.
(c) May be false negative for lesions < 10 mm [17].

References

1. Rare lung cancers. Breathe. 2015;11(4):323–30.
2. NCCN Guidelines Version 7.2015 – Non-Small Cell Lung Cancer.
3. Ost D, Fein AM, Feinsilver SH. Clinical practice. The solitary pulmonary nodule. N Engl J Med. 2003;348(25):2535–42.
4. Burt JR, Iribarren C, Fair JM, Norton LC, Mahbouba M, Rubin GD, et al. Incidental findings on cardiac multidetector row computed tomography among healthy older adults: prevalence and clinical correlates. Arch Intern Med. 2008;168(7):756–61.
5. Wahidi MM, Govert JA, Goudar RK, Gould MK, McCrory DC. Evidence for the treatment of patients with pulmonary nodules: when is it lung cancer?: ACCP evidence-based clinical practice guidelines (2nd edition). Chest. 2007;132(3 Suppl):94S–107S.
6. Deppen S, Putnam JB, Andrade G, Speroff T, Nesbitt JC, Lambright ES, et al. Accuracy of FDG-PET to diagnose lung cancer in a region of endemic granulomatous disease. Ann Thorac Surg. 2011;92(2):428–33.
7. Deppen SA, Blume JD, Kensinger CD, Morgan AM, Aldrich MC, Massion PP, et al. Accuracy of FDG-PET to diagnose lung cancer in areas with infectious lung disease: a meta-analysis. JAMA. 2014;312(12):1227–36.

8. Gould MK, Donington J, Lynch WR, Mazzone PJ, Midthun DE, Naidich DP, et al. Evaluation of individuals with pulmonary nodules: when is it lung cancer? Diagnosis and management of lung cancer, 3rd ed: American College of Chest Physicians evidence-based clinical practice guidelines. Chest. 2013;143(5 Suppl):e93S–120S.

9. Puranik AD, Purandare NC, Shah S, Agrawal A, Rangarajan V. Role of FDG PET/CT in assessing response to targeted therapy in metastatic lung cancers: morphological versus metabolic criteria. Indian J Nucl Med. 2015;30(1):21–5.

10. Mattoli MV, Massaccesi M, Castelluccia A, Scolozzi V, Mantini G, Calcagni ML. The predictive value of 18F-FDG PET-CT for assessing the clinical outcomes in locally advanced NSCLC patients after a new induction treatment: low-dose fractionated radiotherapy with concurrent chemotherapy. Radiat Oncol Lond Engl. 2017;12(1):4.

11. Usmanij EA, Natroshvili T, Timmer-Bonte JNH, Oyen WJG, van der Drift MA, Bussink J, et al. The predictive value of early in-treatment FDG-PET/CT response to chemotherapy in combination with bevacizumab in advanced non-squamous non-small cell lung cancer. J Nucl Med. 2017;58:1243.

12. Goudarzi B, Jacene HA, Wahl RL. Diagnosis and differentiation of bronchioloalveolar carcinoma from adenocarcinoma with bronchioloalveolar components with metabolic and anatomic characteristics using PET/CT. J Nucl Med. 2008;49(10):1585–92.

13. Zhao S, Wu N, Zheng R, Liu Y, Zhang W, Liang Y, et al. Primary tumor SUVmax measured on (18)F-FDG PET-CT correlates with histologic grade and pathologic stage in non-small cell lung cancer. Zhonghua Zhong Liu Za Zhi. 2013;35(10):754–7.

14. Shen G, Lan Y, Zhang K, Ren P, Jia Z. Correction: comparison of 18F-FDG PET/CT and DWI for detection of mediastinal nodal metastasis in non-small cell lung cancer: a meta-analysis. PLoS One. 2017;12(4):e0176150.

15. Hjorthaug K, Hojbjerg JA, Knap MM, Tietze A, Haraldsen A, Zacho HD, et al. Accuracy of 18F-FDG PET-CT in triaging lung cancer patients with suspected brain metastases for MRI. Nucl Med Commun. 2015;36(11):1084–90.

16. Song JW, Oh Y-M, Shim T-S, Kim WS, Ryu J-S, Choi C-M. Efficacy comparison between (18)F-FDG PET/CT and bone scintigraphy in detecting bony metastases of non-small-cell lung cancer. Lung Cancer. 2009;65(3):333–8.

17. Boland GWL, Dwamena BA, Jagtiani Sangwaiya M, Goehler AG, Blake MA, Hahn PF, et al. Characterization of adrenal masses by using FDG PET: a systematic review and meta-analysis of diagnostic test performance. Radiology. 2011;259(1):117–26.

18. Fletcher JW, Kymes SM, Gould M, Alazraki N, Coleman RE, Lowe VJ, et al. A comparison of the diagnostic accuracy of 18F-FDG PET and CT in the characterization of solitary pulmonary nodules. J Nucl Med. 2008;49(2):179–85.

19. Yousefi-Koma A, Panah-Moghaddam M, Kalff V. The utility of metabolic imaging by 18F-FDG PET/CT in lung cancer: impact on diagnosis and staging. Tanaffos. 2013;12(1):16–25.

20. De Leyn P, Dooms C, Kuzdzal J, Lardinois D, Passlick B, Rami-Porta R, et al. Revised ESTS guidelines for preoperative mediastinal lymph node staging for non-small-cell lung cancer. Eur J Cardiothorac Surg. 2014;45(5):787–98.

21. Hara M, Sakurai K, Nakagawa M, Ozawa Y, Shibamoto Y, Tamaki T, et al. The pitfalls of FDG-PET for managing the patients with primary lung cancer. Haigan. 2007;47(2):169–80.

22. Hany TF, Heuberger J, von Schulthess GK. Iatrogenic FDG foci in the lungs: a pitfall of PET image interpretation. Eur Radiol. 2003;13(9):2122–7.

23. Cook GJ, Wegner EA, Fogelman I. Pitfalls and artifacts in 18FDG PET and PET/CT oncologic imaging. Semin Nucl Med. 2004;34(2):122–33.

24. Strauss LG. Fluorine-18 deoxyglucose and false-positive results: a major problem in the diagnostics of oncological patients. Eur J Nucl Med. 1996;23(10):1409–15.

25. Chao F, Zhang H. PET/CT in the staging of the non-small-cell lung cancer. J Biomed Biotechnol. 2012;2012:8.

26. Cheran SK, Nielsen ND, Patz EFJ. False-negative findings for primary lung tumors on FDG positron emission tomography: staging and prognostic implications. AJR Am J Roentgenol. 2004;182(5):1129–32.

27. Bille A, Okiror L, Skanjeti A, Errico L, Arena V, Penna D, et al. Evaluation of integrated positron emission tomography and computed tomography accuracy in detecting lymph node metastasis in patients with adenocarcinoma vs squamous cell carcinoma. Eur J Cardiothorac Surg. 2013;43(3):574–9.
28. Wang Memoli JS, Nietert PJ, Silvestri GA. Meta-analysis of guided bronchoscopy for the evaluation of the pulmonary nodule. Chest. 2012;142(2):385–93.
29. Caroli P, Nanni C, Rubello D, Alavi A, Fanti S. Non-FDG PET in the practice of oncology. Indian J Cancer. 2010;47(2):120–5.
30. Guo W, Hao B, Chen H, Zhao L, Luo Z, Wu H, et al. PET/CT-guided percutaneous biopsy of FDG-avid metastatic bone lesions in patients with advanced lung cancer: a safe and effective technique. Eur J Nucl Med Mol Imaging. 2017;44(1):25–32.
31. Guralnik L, Rozenberg R, Frenkel A, Israel O, Keidar Z. Metabolic PET/CT-guided lung lesion biopsies: impact on diagnostic accuracy and rate of sampling error. J Nucl Med. 2015;56(4):518–22.
32. Taus A, Aguilo R, Curull V, Suarez-Pinera M, Rodriguez-Fuster A, Rodriguez de Dios N, et al. Impact of 18F-FDG PET/CT in the treatment of patients with non-small cell lung cancer. Arch Bronconeumol. 2014;50(3):99–104.
33. Banna GL, Anile G, Russo G, Vigneri P, Castaing M, Nicolosi M, et al. Predictive and prognostic value of early disease progression by PET evaluation in advanced non-small cell lung cancer. Oncology. 2017;92(1):39–47.
34. Liu J, Dong M, Sun X, Li W, Xing L, Yu J. Prognostic value of 18F-FDG PET/CT in surgical non-small cell lung cancer: a meta-analysis. PLoS One. 2016;11(1):e0146195.
35. NCCN Guidelines Version 1.2016 – Small Cell Lung Cancer.
36. Daouk J, Leloire M, Fin L, Bailly P, Morvan J, El Esper I, et al. Respiratory-gated 18F-FDG PET imaging in lung cancer: effects on sensitivity and specificity. Acta Radiol. 2011;52(6):651–7.
37. Nehmeh SA, Erdi YE, Ling CC, Rosenzweig KE, Schoder H, Larson SM, et al. Effect of respiratory gating on quantifying PET images of lung cancer. J Nucl Med. 2002;43(7):876–81.
38. Grootjans W, Hermsen R, van der Heijden EHFM, Schuurbiers-Siebers OCJ, Visser EP, Oyen WJG, et al. The impact of respiratory gated positron emission tomography on clinical staging and management of patients with lung cancer. Lung Cancer. 2015;90(2):217–23.
39. MacManus M, Nestle U, Rosenzweig KE, Carrio I, Messa C, Belohlavek O, et al. Use of PET and PET/CT for radiation therapy planning: IAEA expert report. Radiother Oncol. 2009;91(1):85–94.
40. Shroff GS, Carter BW, Viswanathan C, Benveniste MF, Wu CC, Marom EM, et al. Challenges in interpretation of staging PET/CT in thoracic malignancies. Curr Probl Diagn Radiol. [cited 2017 Jun 2]; Available from: https://doi.org/10.1067/j.cpradiol.2016.11.012
41. Pericleous M, Karpathakis A, Toumpanakis C, Lumgair H, Reiner J, Marelli L, et al. Well-differentiated bronchial neuroendocrine tumors: clinical management and outcomes in 105 patients. Clin Respir J. 2016; https://doi.org/10.1111/crj.12603.
42. Bongiovanni A, Recine F, Riva N, Foca F, Liverani C, Mercatali L, et al. Outcome analysis of first-line somatostatin analog treatment in metastatic pulmonary neuroendocrine tumors and prognostic significance of 18FDG-PET/CT. Clin Lung Cancer. 2016; https://doi.org/10.1016/j.cllc.2016.11.004.
43. Uhlen N, Grundberg O, Jacobsson H, Sundin A, Dobra K, Sanchez-Crespo A, et al. 18F-FDG PET/CT diagnosis of bronchopulmonary carcinoids versus pulmonary hamartomas. Clin Nucl Med. 2016;41(4):263–7.
44. Bradley J, Bae K, Choi N, Forster K, Siegel BA, Brunetti J, et al. A phase II comparative study of gross tumor volume definition with or without PET/CT fusion in Dosimetric planning for non-small cell lung cancer (NSCLC): primary analysis of Radiation Therapy Oncology Group (RTOG) 0515. Int J Radiat Oncol Biol Phys. 2012;82(1):435–441.e1.

45. Nestle U, Kremp S, Grosu A-L. Practical integration of [18F]-FDG-PET and PET-CT in the planning of radiotherapy for non-small cell lung cancer (NSCLC): the technical basis, ICRU-target volumes, problems, perspectives. Radiother Oncol. 2006;81(2):209–25.
46. Gould MK, Sanders GD, Barnett PG, Rydzak CE, Maclean CC, McClellan MB, et al. Cost-effectiveness of alternative management strategies for patients with solitary pulmonary nodules. Ann Intern Med. 2003;138(9):724–35.
47. Lejeune C, Al Zahouri K, Woronoff-Lemsi M-C, Arveux P, Bernard A, Binquet C, et al. Use of a decision analysis model to assess the medicoeconomic implications of FDG PET imaging in diagnosing a solitary pulmonary nodule. Eur J Health Econ. 2005;6(3):203–14.

Bibliography & Further Reading

Evidence-based indications for the use of PET-CT in the United Kingdom 2022
The Royal College of Radiologists, Royal College of Physicians, British Nuclear
Medicine Society, Administration of Radioactive Substances Advisory Committee
www.rcr.ac.uk

1. What are the common indications of ^{18}F-fluorodeoxyglucose (18F-FDG) positron emission tomography (PET)-computed tomography (CT) in breast cancer?

   Common indications of 18F-FDG PET-CT in breast cancer include the following:

   (a) Staging—detection of metastases
   (b) Treatment response evaluation
   (c) Detection of recurrence and restaging [1]
   (d) Assess indeterminate or equivocal breast lesions

2. What is the role of 18F-FDG PET-CT in diagnosing primary breast cancer?

   Despite relatively high specificity, 18F-FDG PET-CT is not routinely used in the diagnosis of early-stage breast cancer due to its poor spatial resolution and resultant low sensitivity. Mammography, ultrasonography, and magnetic resonance imaging (MRI) are the modalities of choice for the primary diagnosis of breast cancer. Positron emission mammography, an emerging modality, has higher spatial resolution and may be a valuable tool in primary breast cancer diagnostics, particularly in cases where conventional modalities have limited accuracy (e.g., dense breast) [2–4].

3. What is the role of 18F-FDG PET-CT in staging of breast cancer?

   18F-FDG PET-CT has limited accuracy in T and N staging of breast cancer when compared to MRI and sentinel lymph node biopsy, respectively. However, 18F-FDG PET-CT is useful in the identification of extra axillary lymph nodal and distant metastases, particularly in patients with locally advanced breast cancer, where the prevalence of metastases is high [1, 5].

4. What is the role of 18F-FDG PET-CT in the re-staging of breast cancer?

   18F-FDG PET-CT is useful in detecting recurrent disease in breast cancer with a sensitivity and specificity of around 90% [1, 6–8].

© The Author(s), under exclusive license to Springer Nature
Switzerland AG 2026
S. Raja et al., *Question and Answers in PET/CT*,
https://doi.org/10.1007/978-3-032-00821-3_6

5. What is the role of 18F-FDG PET-CT in the assessment of treatment response in breast cancer?

    18F-FDG PET-CT may be applicable for response evaluation of neoadjuvant chemotherapy, with a meta-analysis showing pooled sensitivity and specificity of 84% and 71% for predicting pathological response. Even though 18F-FDG PET-CT is accurate in evaluating lytic and mixed bone metastases, its diagnostic performance in osteoblastic bone metastases is limited, as they frequently do not show increased FDG uptake.

    Following hormonotherapy, there may be a transient increase in glucose uptake despite an eventual favorable response, known as the metabolic flare phenomenon [5, 9–11].

6. What are the sensitivity and specificity of 18F-FDG PET-CT in detecting breast cancers?

    Although the specificity of FDG-PET/CT is moderately high in the primary diagnosis of breast cancer (ranging from 73% to 100%), the sensitivity is low (ranging from 48% to 96%), mainly due to its low spatial resolution [12].

7. What are the sensitivity and specificity of 18F-FDG PET-CT in the assessment of nodal disease in breast cancer?

    A meta-analysis showed that 18F-FDG PET-CT has a low pooled sensitivity of 63% with a high specificity of 94% in detecting axillary lymph nodal metastases in breast cancer [13].

8. What are the sensitivity and specificity of 18F-FDG PET-CT in the assessment of distant metastasis?

    A meta-analysis showed 96% and 95% sensitivity and specificity for 18-F FDG-PET/CT in detecting distant metastases in breast cancer [14].

9. What is the role of 18F-FDG PET-CT in T staging?

    The accuracy of conventional 18F-FDG PET-CT in T staging of breast cancer is limited when compared to MRI. However, PET CT mammography, which is acquired with a patient in a prone position using a special breast-positioning aid, shows almost similar accuracy in T staging compared to MR mammography and seems more accurate than MRI in revealing the focality of disease [15, 16].

10. What is the role of 18F-FDG PET-CT in N staging?

    18F-FDG PET-CT is not useful in routine assessment of axillary lymph nodal metastases, particularly in early-stage breast cancers, where sentinel lymph node biopsy is the standard of care. However, it helps detect extra-axillary lymph nodal metastases, significantly impacting management [5, 17, 18].

11. What is the role of 18F-FDG PET-CT in M staging?

    18F-FDG PET-CT is beneficial in detecting distant metastases with more than 95% accuracy, mainly when locally advanced breast cancer is present or lymph nodes are palpable [14, 19, 20].

12. What is the role of 18F-FDG PET-CT in the assessment of skeletal metastases?

Even though 18F-FDG-PET/CT is highly accurate in identifying lytic mar-row (invisible on CT) and mixed bone metastases, it lacks sensitivity in the detection of osteoblastic metastases (where bone scan seems to be more sensi-tive at the cost of poor specificity and lower sensitivity for lytic metastases). A meta-analysis showed better accuracy for MRI (sensitivity and specificity of 97%) in detecting bone metastases when compared to PET (sensitivity and specificity of 83% and 95%, respectively) [1, 21, 22].

13. What are the common pitfalls of 18F-FDG PET-CT in breast cancer?

Increased FDG uptake may be seen in various benign conditions such as fibroadenomas, gynecomastia, fat necrosis, and inflammatory conditions. FDG uptake may be low or absent in small lesions and in a few tumor subtypes such as lobular carcinoma, mucinous carcinoma, carcinoma in situ, or slow-growing tumors like tubular carcinoma.

Following hormonotherapy, a transient increase in glucose uptake can occur despite a favorable response, known as the metabolic flare phenomenon [1, 5, 11, 23–26].

14. What are the common false-positive 18F-FDG PET-CT findings in breast cancer?

Common false-positive 18F-FDG PET-CT findings in breast cancer are as follows:

(a) FDG uptake in various benign conditions such as fibroadenomas, ductal hyperplasia, gynecomastia, fat necrosis, silicone granuloma, and inflam-matory/infective conditions such as mastitis, sarcoidosis, tuberculosis, and so on

(b) Treatment-related changes such as post-surgery (e.g., seroma, hematoma) or radiotherapy inflammatory changes

(c) Flare phenomenon following hormonotherapy/chemotherapy

(d) In addition, various artifacts such as misregistration, partial volume effect, attenuation correction, and truncation artifacts can result in false positives [1, 5, 24–27].

15. What are the common false-negative 18F-FDG PET-CT findings in breast cancer?

Common false-negative 18F-FDG PET-CT findings in breast cancer are as follows:

(a) Tumor subtypes such as lobular carcinoma, mucinous carcinoma, carci-noma in situ, or slow-growing tumors like tubular carcinoma, as well as necrotic lesions, may show lower or negligible FDG uptake

(b) Small-sized lesions/lymph nodes (smaller than the resolution of PET scanner)

(c) Post-chemotherapy status

(d) Artifacts such as misregistration artifacts [25–27]

16. What are non-FDG PET tracers used in imaging of breast cancer?
    Non-FDG PET tracers used in imaging of breast cancer include the following:

    (a) Estrogen receptor imaging—[18F] fluoro-17β-estradiol
    (b) Progesterone   receptor   imaging—18F-Fluorofuranylnorprogesterone (FFNP)
    (c) HER2 receptor imaging—89Zr (64Cu/68 Ga)-Trastuzumab
    (d) Proliferation tracer—18F-FLT
    (e) Membrane lipids imaging—11C or 18F-labeled choline
    (f) Amino acid transport—11C-methionine [28]

17. What is the prognostic value of FDG uptake in the primary tumor?
    The intensity of FDG uptake and its semi-quantitative parameter SUV Max seems to predict prognosis in early-stage as well as metastatic breast cancer, as patients with low SUV Max have a better prognosis [10, 29–31].

18. What is the role of 18F-FDG PET-CT in radiotherapy planning in breast cancer?
    18F-FDG PET-CT may be useful in the radiotherapy planning of breast cancer by identifying additional sites of disease, particularly extra-axillary lymph nodal (internal mammary or supraclavicular) and distant metastatic sites. It may also show subregions or foci with increased or altered biologic activity within the gross tumor volume that could be preferentially targeted and treated with escalated radiation doses [32–34].

19. What is the cost-effectiveness of 18F-FDG PET-CT in breast cancer?
    Even though 18F-FDG PET-CT seems to be a cost-effective investigation in the detection of distant metastases in breast cancer, only limited data is available on the cost effectiveness of 18F-FDG PET-CT in various indications of breast cancer [35–37].

20. What are the advantages and limitations of 18F-FDG PET-CT in breast cancer?
    Advantages: 18F-FDG PET-CT is useful in detecting distant metastases and recurrences in patients with breast cancer. It may also help assess treatment response evaluation.
    Limitations: 18F-FDG PET-CT is not useful in primary diagnosis and axillary lymph nodal breast cancer staging. Its sensitivity is limited to a few subtypes of breast cancer such as lobular carcinoma, tubular carcinoma, mucinous carcinoma, and so on, as well as in detecting brain and sclerotic bone metastases [1, 2, 5].

References

1. Hildebrandt MG, Kodahl AR, Teilmann-Jørgensen D, Mogensen O, Jensen PT. [18F]fluorode-oxyglucose PET/computed tomography in breast cancer and gynecologic cancers: a literature review. PET Clin. 2015;10(1):89–104.
2. Warning K, Hildebrandt MG, Kristensen B, Ewertz M. Utility of 18FDG-PET/CT in breast cancer diagnostics–a systematic review. Dan Med Bull. 2011;58(7):A4289.

3. Moadel RM. Breast cancer imaging devices. Semin Nucl Med. 2011;41(3):229–41.
4. Surti S. Radionuclide methods and instrumentation for breast cancer detection and diagnosis. Semin Nucl Med. 2013;43(4):271–80.
5. Vercher-Conejero JL, Pelegrí-Martinez L, Lopez-Aznar D, del Cózar-Santiago MP. Positron emission tomography in breast cancer. Diagnostics (Basel). 2015;5(1):61–83.
6. Pennant M, Takwoingi Y, Pennant L, et al. A systematic review of positron emission tomography (PET) and positron emission tomography/computed tomography (PET/CT) for the diagnosis of breast cancer recurrence. Health Technol Assess. 2010;14(50):1–103.
7. Schneble EJ, Graham LJ, Shupe MP, et al. Future directions for the early detection of recurrent breast cancer. J Cancer. 2014;5(4):291–300.
8. Champion L, Brain E, Giraudet AL, et al. Breast cancer recurrence diagnosis suspected on tumor marker rising: value of whole-body 18FDG-PET/CT imaging and impact on patient management. Cancer. 2011;117(8):1621–9.
9. Cheng X, Li Y, Liu B, Xu Z, Bao L, Wang J. 18F-FDG PET/CT and PET for evaluation of pathological response to neoadjuvant chemotherapy in breast cancer: a meta-analysis. Acta Radiol. 2012;53(6):615–27.
10. Morris PG, Ulaner GA, Eaton A, et al. Standardized uptake value by positron emission tomography/computed tomography as a prognostic variable in metastatic breast cancer. Cancer. 2012;118:5454–62.
11. Mortimer JE, Dehdashti F, Siegel BA, Trinkaus K, Katzenellenbogen JA, Welch MJ. Metabolic flare: indicator of hormone responsiveness in advanced breast cancer. J Clin Oncol. 2001;19:2797–803.
12. Warning K, Hildebrandt MG, Kristensen B, et al. Utility of 18FDG-PET/CT in breast cancer diagnostics–a systematic review. Dan Med Bull. 2011;58(7):A4289.
13. Cooper KL, Harnan S, Meng Y, et al. Positron emission tomography (PET) for assessment of axillary lymph node status in early breast cancer: a systematic review and meta-analysis. Eur J Surg Oncol. 2011;37(3):187–98.
14. Hong S, Li J, Wang S. 18FDG PET-CT for diagnosis of distant metastases in breast cancer patients. A meta-analysis. Surg Oncol. 2013;22(2):139–43.
15. Heusner TA, Kuemmel S, Umutlu L, et al. Breast cancer staging in a single session: whole-body PET/CT mammography. J Nucl Med. 2008;49(8):1215–22.
16. Moon EH, Lim ST, Han YH, et al. The usefulness of F-18 FDG PET/CT-mammography for preoperative staging of breast cancer: comparison with conventional PET/CT and MR-mammography. Radiol Oncol. 2013;47(4):390–7.
17. Riegger C, Koeninger A, Hartung V, et al. Comparison of the diagnostic value of FDG-PET/CT and axillary ultrasound for the detection of lymph node metastases in breast cancer patients. Acta Radiol. 2012;53:1092–8.
18. Aukema TS, Straver ME, Peeters MJ, et al. Detection of extra-axillary lymph node involvement with FDG PET/CT in patients with stage II–III breast cancer. Eur J Cancer. 2010;46:3205–10.
19. Groheux D, Giacchetti S, Delord M, et al. 18F-FDG PET/CT in staging patients with locally advanced or inflammatory breast cancer: comparison to conventional staging. J Nucl Med. 2013;54:5–11.
20. Pan L, Han Y, Sun X, et al. FDG-PET and other imaging modalities for the evaluation of breast cancer recurrence and metastases: a meta-analysis. J Cancer Res Clin Oncol. 2010;136(7):1007–22.
21. Liu T, Cheng T, Xu W, et al. A meta-analysis of 18FDG-PET, MRI and bone scintigraphy for diagnosis of bone metastases in patients with breast cancer. Skeletal Radiol. 2011;40(5):523–31.
22. Evangelista L, Panunzio A, Polverosi R, et al. Early bone marrow metastasis detection: the additional value of FDG-PET/CT vs. CT Imaging Biomed Pharmacother. 2012;66(6):448–53.
23. Kumar R, Chauhan A, Zhuang H, Chandra P, Schnall M, Alavi A. Clinicopathologic factors associated with false negative FDG-PET in primary breast cancer. Breast Cancer Res Treat. 2006;98:267–74.
24. Adejolu M, Huo L, Rohren E, Santiago L, Yang WT. False-positive lesions mimicking breast cancer on FDG PET and PET/CT. Am J Roentgenol. 2012;198(3):W304–14.

25. Dong A, Wang Y, Lu J, Zuo C. Spectrum of the breast lesions with increased 18F-FDG uptake on PET/CT. Clin Nucl Med. 2016;41(7):543–57.
26. Kumar R, Rani N, Patel C, Basu S, Alavi A. False-negative and false-positive results in FDG-PET and PET/CT in breast cancer. PET Clin. 2009;4(3):289–98.
27. Corrigan AJ, Schleyer PJ, Cook GJ. Pitfalls and artifacts in the use of PET/CT in oncology imaging. Semin Nucl Med. 2015;45(6):481–99.
28. Linden HM, Dehdashti F. Novel methods and tracers for breast cancer imaging. Semin Nucl Med. 2013;43(4):324–9.
29. Ekmekcioglu O, Aliyev A, Yilmaz S, et al. Correlation of 18F-fluorodeoxyglucose uptake with histopathological prognostic factors in breast carcinoma. Nucl Med Commun. 2013;34:1055–67.
30. Murakami R, FukushimaY TH, et al. Prognostic value of SUVmax of 18F-FDG PET/CT in early stage breast cancer with no LN metastasis. Open J Med Imaging. 2017;7:112–23.
31. Cokmert S, Tanriverdi O, Karapolat I, et al. The maximum standardized uptake value of meta-static site in 18 F-FDG PET/CT predicts molecular subtypes and survival in metastatic breast cancer: an Izmir Oncology Group study. J BUON. 2016;21(6):1410–8.
32. Gunalp B, Ince S, Karacalioglu AO, Ayan A, Emer O, Alagoz E. Clinical impact of (18) F-FDG PET/CT on initial staging and therapy planning for breast cancer. Exp Ther Med. 2012;4(4):693–8.
33. Beriwal S. PET/CT in radiation therapy planning for breast cancer. PET Clin. 2009;4(4):349–57.
34. Heron DE, Beriwal S, Avril N. FDG-PET and PET/CT in radiation therapy simulation and man-agement of patients who have primary and recurrent breast cancer. PET Clin. 2006;1(1):39–49.
35. Miquel-Cases A, Teixeira S, Retèl V, et al. Cost-effectiveness of 18f-Fdg pet/Ct for screening distant metastasis in stage ii/iii breast cancer patients of the UK, the United States and The Netherlands. Value Health. 2015;18(7):A337.
36. Sloka JS, Hollett PD, Mathews M. Cost-effectiveness of positron emission tomography in breast cancer. Mol Imaging Biol. 2005;7:351–60.
37. Annunziata S, Caldarella C, Treglia G. Cost-effectiveness of Fluorine-18-Fluorodeoxyglucose positron emission tomography in tumours other than lung cancer: a systematic review. World J Radiol. 2014;6(3):48–55.

Colorectal Cancer

7

1. What are the common histological types of colorectal cancer (CRC)?
   (a) Adenocarcinoma (most common type; including mucinous carcinoma and signet ring cell carcinoma) [1]
   (b) Neuroendocrine tumors (carcinoid)
   (c) Adenosquamous carcinoma
   (d) Spindle cell carcinoma
   (e) Undifferentiated carcinoma

2. What are the common indications of ^{18}F-fluorodeoxyglucose (18F-FDG) positron emission tomography (PET)-computed tomography (CT) in CRC?
   A. Response assessment after neoadjuvant therapy or palliative therapy
   B. Detection of recurrent disease
   C. Radiotherapy planning [1, 2]
   D. Staging of patients with synchronous metastases at presentation suitable for resection or patients with equivocal findings on other imaging

3. What is the role of 18F-FDG PET in diagnosing CRC?
   18F FDG PET/CT is not routinely recommended to diagnose CRC or as a screening test. This is mainly due to high and variable physiological FDG uptake in the colon and its inability to distinguish benign (adenomas) and malignant colonic lesions [2].

4. What is the role of 18F-FDG PET in staging CRC?
   18F FDG PET/CT is not routinely used in the staging of CRC. The primary indication of FDG PET/CT in preoperative cases of CRC is an assessment of indeterminate lesions on conventional imaging before metastatectomy. FDG PET/CT may change the treatment protocol in up to 30% of CRC patients [3, 4].

S. Raja et al., *Question and Answers in PET/CT*,
https://doi.org/10.1007/978-3-032-00821-3_7

5. What is the role of 18F-FDG PET in the assessment of CRC recurrence?

    FDG PET/CT is beneficial and superior to conventional imaging in evaluating the recurrence of CRC in patients with rising carcinoembryonic antigen (CEA) levels [5].

6. What is the role of 18F-FDG PET in the assessment of treatment response in CRC?

    FDG PET/CT is beneficial and superior to conventional endoscopic ultrasound in the response assessment of neoadjuvant therapy for rectal cancer patients. FDG PET/CT is also valuable for evaluating targeted therapies (such as Transarterial Chemoembolization (TACE), Transarterial Radioembolization (TARE), and Radiofrequency Ablation (RFA)) in patients with unresectable colorectal liver metastases [5–7].

7. What are the sensitivity, specificity, positive likelihood ratio, and negative likelihood ratio of 18F-FDG in CRCs?

    FDG PET/CT is useful in identifying the colorectal primary tumor and correctly classifying the T stage with an accuracy of 94% [8].

    The sensitivity, specificity, positive likelihood ratio, and negative likelihood ratio of FDG PET/CT in detecting pre-therapeutic lymph node involvement in patients with CRC were 42.9%, 87.9%, 2.82, and 0.69, respectively [9].

8. What are the sensitivity and specificity of 18F-FDG in the assessment of distant metastasis?

    The sensitivity and specificity of 18F-FDG PET/CT in detecting colorectal liver metastases per patient are 96.5% and 97.2%, respectively [10].

    The sensitivity and specificity of 18F-FDG PET/CT in detecting colorectal extrahepatic metastases are 75–89% and 95–96%, respectively [11].

9. What is the role of 18F-FDG PET-CT in T staging?

    FDG PET/CT is an accurate modality for identifying primary tumors and defining the local extent of CRC, which is particularly useful in radiotherapy planning of rectal cancer. However, detecting smaller tumors by FDG PET CT is not optimal, and the distinction between adenoma and carcinoma cannot be made reliably [12].

10. What is the role of 18F-FDG PET-CT in N staging?

    Although the specificity of 18F-FDG PET-CT is high in detecting colorectal lymph nodal metastases, sensitivity is low, which might be due to insufficient spatial resolution of the PET scanner for small-sized lymph nodes and obscuring of nodes by physiologic activity in the intestine and urinary bladder, or by the nearby primary tumor. So, as of now, there is no solid evidence to support the routine clinical application of PET/CT in evaluating lymph node status in patients with CRC [12].

11. What is the role of 18F-FDG PET-CT in M staging?

FDG PET/CT is very sensitive and specific in detecting colorectal and hepatic metastases. However, it is not superior to Contrast-Enhanced Computed Tomograph (CECT) and magnetic resonance imaging (MRI) (MRI being more sensitive in detecting smaller lesions), which are first-line investigations. However, when CT or MRI is doubtful, PET/CT should be used as a second-line investigation to evaluate hepatic metastases [12].

12. What are the sensitivity and specificity of 18F-FDG PET in the assessment of CRC recurrence?

The sensitivity and specificity of 18F-FDG PET in detecting tumor recurrence in CRC patients are 90.3% and 80.0% [13].

13. What are the common pitfalls of 18F-FDG PET-CT in CRC?

Common pitfalls of 18F-FDG PET-CT in CRC include the following:

(a) Physiological variants in FDG uptake in bowel (ranging from no discernible uptake above background to diffuse intense FDG uptake)
(b) Technical artifacts due to misregistration, partial volume effect, attenuation correction, and truncation effect
(c) Pathology-specific pitfalls in various organs such as urinary activity and uptake in reproductive uptake, and so on
(d) Treatment-related pitfalls due to surgery, chemotherapy, radiotherapy, and exogenous marrow stimulation [14]

14. What are the common false-positive 18F-FDG PET-CT findings in CRC?

Common false-positive 18F-FDG PET-CT findings include infection/inflammatory conditions, urinary tracer activity, physiological uptake in the reproductive system, treatment-related changes like hematoma, post-radiotherapy inflammation, chemotherapy-induced lung changes, and so on; in addition, various artifacts such as misregistration artifact, partial volume effect, attenuation correction artifact, and truncation artifact can result in false positives [14].

15. What are the common false-negative 18F-FDG PET-CT findings in CRC?

Common false-negative 18F-FDG PET-CT findings in CRC are as follows:

(a) Small-sized lesions/lymph nodes (smaller than the resolution of PET scanner)
(b) Mucinous adenocarcinomas
(c) Post-chemotherapy status
(d) Artifacts like misregistration artifact [14]

16. What are non-FDG tracers in imaging CRC?

(a) Proliferative marker—for example, F-18 fluorothymidine
(b) Hypoxia agents—for example, F-18 fluoromisonidasole
(c) Somatostatin analogs–for example, Ga-68 DOTA-tyrosine3-octreotate (DOTATATE) (for neuroendocrine tumors)
(d) Anti-CEA monoclonal antibody imaging—Tc-99m Arcitumomab [15, 16]

17. What is the role of 18F-FDG PET-CT in the management of CRC?

In the initial evaluation of CRCs, FDG PET/CT plays a vital role in indeterminate liver lesions detected on CT/ MRI and in detecting extrahepatic metastatic disease, particularly locally advanced CRCs. FDG PET/CT may help assess the treatment response of CRC. FDG PET/CT has a definite role in the assessment of suspected CRC recurrence during follow-up. FDG PET/CT is useful in radiotherapy planning of rectal cancers [12].

18. What is the role of 18F-FDG PET-CT in radiotherapy planning in CRC?

Recent studies show that FDG PET/CT improves standardization of tumor target volume delineation in rectal cancer and helps to minimize the radiation dose to surrounding normal structures and consequently reduce radiotherapy-induced morbidity [15].

19. What are the limitations of 18F-FDG PET-CT in radiotherapy planning?

Several methods (percentage of maximum SUV, fixed SUV cut-off of 2.5, confidence-connected region-growing method, etc.) are being used for tumor volume segmentation. However, the optimal method for tumor volume segmentation is yet to be standardized. Even though initial studies have shown that FDG PET/CT has better accuracy and low inter-observer variability for determining tumor target volume of rectal cancer, its advantage over the standard technique CT (already in practice) has not been proven in terms of patient outcome [17].

20. What are the advantages and limitations of FDG PET-CT in CRC?

Advantages:
(a) Very useful in the assessment of distant metastases, particularly in the characterization of indeterminate liver lesions detected on CT/MRI
(b) Most sensitive investigation in detecting recurrent disease
(c) Emerging role in therapy response assessment and radiotherapy planning of rectal cancer [12]

Limitations:
(a) Nonspecific nature of the tracer with various false-positive findings (although careful interpretation may identify most of them)
(b) FDG avidity is low in a few tumor subtypes such as mucinous tumors and well-differentiated neuroendocrine tumors
(c) More research is required for indications such as therapy response assessment and radiotherapy planning
(d) Lack of standardization of methods used for tumor volume segmentation in radiotherapy planning
(e) Relatively high cost
(f) Radiation exposure [12, 17]

References

1. Cotran RS, Kumar V, Fausto N, Fausto N, Robbins SL, Abbas AK. Robbins and Cotran pathologic basis of disease. 7th ed. St. Louis: Elsevier Saunders; 2005. p. 864.
2. Vikram R, Iyer RB. PET/CT imaging in the diagnosis, staging, and follow-up of colorectal cancer. Cancer Imaging. 2008;8:S46–51.
3. Davey K, Heriot AG, Mackay J, et al. The impact of 18-fluorodexoyglucose positron emission tomography-computed tomography on the staging and management of primary rectal cancer. Dis Colon Rectum. 2008;51:9971003.
4. Petersen R, Hess S, Alavi A, Carlsen PH. FDG-PET/CT for initial staging of colorectal cancer. J Nucl Med. 2014;55(Suppl):1556.
5. Agarwal A, Marcus C, Xiao J, Nene P, Kachnic LA, Subramaniam RM. FDG PET/CT in the management of colorectal and anal cancers. Am J Roentgenol. 2014;203:1109–19.
6. Amthauer H, Denecke T, Rau B, et al. Response prediction by FDG-PET after neoadjuvant radiochemotherapy and combined regional hyperthermia of rectal cancer: correlation with endorectal ultrasound and histopathology. Eur J Nucl Med Mol Imaging. 2004;31:811–9.
7. Hipps D, Ausania F, Manas DM, Rose JD, French JJ. Selective interarterial radiation therapy (SIRT) in colorectal liver metastases: how do we monitor response? HPB Surg. 2013;2013:570808.
8. Mainenti PP, Iodice D, Segreto S, et al. Colorectal cancer and 18FDG-PET/CT: what about adding the T to the N parameter in loco-regional staging? World J Gastroenterol. 2011;17:1427–33.
9. Lu YY, Chen JH, Ding HJ, et al. A systematic review and meta-analysis of pretherapeutic lymph node staging of colorectal cancer by 18F-FDG PET or PET/CT. Nucl Med Commun. 2012;33:1127–33.
10. Niekel MC, Bipat S, Stoker J. Diagnostic imaging of colorectal liver metastases with CT, MR imaging, FDG PET, and/or FDG PET/CT: a meta-analysis of prospective studies including patients who have not previously undergone treatment. Radiology. 2010;257:674–84.
11. Patel S, McCall M, Ohinmaa A, et al. Positron emission tomography/computed tomographic scans compared to computed tomographic scans for detecting colorectal liver metastases: a systematic review. Ann Surg. 2011;253:666–71.
12. Donswijk ML, Hess S, Mulders T, Lam MG. 18F Fluorodeoxyglucose PET/computed tomography in gastrointestinal malignancies. PET Clin. 2014;9:421–41.
13. Lu YY, Chen JH, Chien CR, et al. Use of FDG-PET or PET/CT to detect recurrent colorectal cancer in patients with elevated CEA: a systematic review and meta-analysis. Int J Color Dis. 2013;28(8):1039–47.
14. Sasikumar A, Joy A. 18F-FDG PET/CT: normal variants, artefacts, and pitfalls in colorectal cancer. In: PET/CT in colorectal cancer; 2017. p. 27–48.
15. Chowdhury FU, Shah N, Scarsbrook AF, Bradley KM. ^{18}F-FDG PET/CT imaging of colorectal cancer: a pictorial review. Postgrad Med J. 2010;86:174–82.
16. Fuster D, Maurel J, Muxí A, et al. Is there a role for (99m)Tc-anti-CEA monoclonal antibody imaging in the diagnosis of recurrent colorectal carcinoma? Q J Nucl Med. 2003;47:109–15.
17. Wang YY, Zhe H. Clinical application of multimodality imaging in radiotherapy treatment planning for rectal cancer. Cancer Imaging. 2013;13:495.

Malignant Melanoma

1. What are the common indications of ^{18}F-fluorodeoxyglucose (18F-FDG) positron emission tomography (PET)-computed tomography (CT) in malignant melanoma?

   Common indications for 18F-FDG PET-CT in malignant melanoma are initial staging (particularly in assessing the distant metastases) and surveillance [1, 2].

2. What is the role of 18F-FDG PET in staging malignant melanoma?

   18F-FDG PET-CT is useful in initial staging, particularly in detecting distant metastases in advanced melanoma patients (i.e., American Joint Committee on Cancer (AJCC) stages III and IV). Its use is very limited in assessing primary site and lymph nodal metastases, and in early malignant melanoma patients, a sentinel lymph node biopsy may be better [1–3].

3. What is the role of 18F-FDG PET in re-staging malignant melanoma?

   18F-FDG PET-CT is useful in detecting metastases during restaging. However, the sensitivity of 18F-FDG PET-CT is lower in detecting local and lymph nodal recurrence, which is better evaluated with ultrasound [2].

4. What is the role of 18F-FDG PET in the assessment of treatment response in malignant melanoma?

   Some studies show that 18F-FDG PET-CT is useful in assessing the response to conventional therapies such as surgery and chemotherapy and in mutation-driven therapy (e.g., vemurafenib and dabrafenib).

   Its use in assessing response to isolated limb chemo infusion is limited because in-transit and satellite metastases may be smaller than PET's resolution. An isolated limb infusion is known to cause regional fat and muscle necrosis, which may result in false positives.

S. Raja et al., *Question and Answers in PET/CT*, https://doi.org/10.1007/978-3-032-00821-3_8

Since immunomodulation is a relatively new treatment modality for melanoma, the role of 18F-FDG PET-CT in its response assessment is yet to be studied. However, there are various challenges/confounding factors for 18F-FDG PET-CT in this patient group, such as pseudoprogression, treatment-induced inflammation, and adverse immune-related reactions following immune modulatory therapy [4–8].

5. What are the sensitivity and specificity of 18F-FDG PET/CT in the assessment of lymph nodal metastasis?

The median sensitivity and specificity of FDG-PET/CT for regional lymph node staging of malignant melanoma are 11% and 97%, respectively [2].

6. What are the sensitivity and specificity of 18F-FDG PET/CT in the assessment of distant metastasis?

The sensitivity and specificity of 18F-FDG PET-CT for detecting distant metastases are 86% and 91%, respectively [2].

7. What is the role of 18F-FDG PET-CT in T staging?

8. 18F-FDG-PET/CT is not helpful in T staging of malignant melanoma since its accuracy in evaluating depth and/or ulceration of primary lesion is less, and these are in the realm of millimeters, below PET resolution. Although the primary lesion is sometimes visualized on PET/CT, this is rarely impactful because the diagnosis is already established [9].

9. What is the role of 18F-FDG PET-CT in N staging?

Even though 18F-FDG PET-CT is highly specific, it is not clinically useful in evaluating regional lymph node basins in patients with newly diagnosed melanoma because of its very low sensitivity. Sentinel lymph node biopsy and ultrasonography play major roles in assessing lymph nodal metastases [2, 8, 9].

10. What is the role of 18F-FDG PET-CT in M staging?

18F-FDG PET-CT is useful in detecting distant metastases in malignant melanoma with the highest accuracy among available techniques, except for brain metastases, where magnetic resonance imaging would be more sensitive [2, 10].

11. What are the common pitfalls of 18F-FDG PET-CT in malignant melanoma?

18F-FDG PET-CT is not a very sensitive procedure in evaluating primary lesions and identifying micrometastases in lymph nodes.

Its role in the treatment response assessment is yet to be proven, particularly following immunomodulation therapies [8].

12. What are the common false-positive 18F-FDG PET-CT findings in malignant melanoma?

Common false-positive PET-CT findings in malignant melanoma are as follows:

(a) Infection/inflammation
(b) Regional fat and muscle necrosis following isolated limb infusion

(c) Immunomodulation therapy-induced inflammation and adverse immune-related reactions such as colitis, dermatitis, hypophysitis, arthritis, and thyroiditis

(d) Pseudoprogression from immunomodulation therapy

(e) Post-operative changes

(f) In addition, various artifacts such as misregistration artifact, partial volume effect, attenuation correction artifact, and truncation artifact can result in false positives [8, 11].

13. What are the common false-negative 18F-FDG PET-CT findings in malignant melanoma?

The common false-negative findings in malignant melanoma are as follows:

(a) Early-stage primary lesions may not be visible on PET/CT

(b) Small-sized lymph nodes/metastatic lesions (smaller than the resolution of the PET scanner)

(c) Post-chemotherapy status

(d) Artifacts like misregistration artifacts, etc. [11]

14. What are non-FDG tracers in imaging malignant melanoma?

No PET tracers other than 18F-FDG are used for imaging malignant melanoma in routine clinical practice. However, as part of the research, the following tracers have been tried, mainly with murine models.

(a) 18F-Fluorothymidine (FLT) (proliferation marker)

(b) 18F-Fluoromisonidazole (FMISO) (hypoxia tracer)

(c) 18F-galacto-RGD/68Ga-Dodecanetetraacetic   acid   (DOTA)-Arginylglycylaspartic acid (RGD) (neoangiogenesis marker)

(d) 18F-Fluro-dihydroxyphenylalanine   (FDOPA)   (targeting   melanin formation)

(e) 64Cu-DOTA-NAPamide (targeting a-melanocyte stimulating hormone)

(f) 64Cu-SarAr (monoclonal antibody against melanoma-associated antigen) [12]

15. What is the role of 18F-FDG PET-CT in radiotherapy planning in malignant melanoma?

Radiotherapy is not routinely used to treat malignant melanomas arising from skin or mucous membranes, where surgery and systemic therapies are the mainstay of treatment. In contrast, radiotherapy is a potential treatment option for treating ocular melanomas to preserve vision, particularly for medium-sized lesions. However, the role of 18F-FDG PET-CT in radiotherapy planning of ocular or other melanomas is yet to be studied [13].

16. What is the cost-effectiveness of 18F-FDG PET-CT in malignant melanoma?

18F-FDG PET-CT seems to be a cost-effective and more accurate investigation in the setting of identifying distant metastases in patients with high-risk malignant melanoma, particularly by avoiding unnecessary surgeries and complications [14].

17. What are the advantages and limitations of 18F-FDG PET-CT in malignant melanoma?

The advantage of 18F-FDG PET-CT in malignant melanoma is its highest sensitivity and specificity among available imaging techniques in detecting distant metastases in advanced melanoma patients (i.e., AJCC stages III and IV).

Limitations of 18F-FDG PET-CT are poor sensitivity in detecting small regional lymph nodal metastases, limited known role in treatment response assessment, and non-specific nature of tracer leading to false-positive findings in infection/inflammation [2, 8].

References

1. Krug B, Crott R, Lonneux M, et al. Role of PET in the initial staging of cutaneous malignant melanoma: systematic review. Radiology. 2008;249(3):836–44.
2. Xing Y, Bronstein Y, Ross MI, et al. Contemporary diagnostic imaging modalities for the staging and surveillance of melanoma patients: a metaanalysis. J Natl Cancer Inst. 2011;103(2):129–42.
3. Karakousis GC, Czerniecki BJ. Diagnosis of Melanoma. PET Clin. 2011 Jan;6:1–8.
4. Strobel K, Skalsky J, Steinert HC, et al. S-100B and FDG-PET/CT in therapy response assessment of melanoma patients. Dermatology. 2007;215:192–201.
5. Beasley GM, Parsons C, Broadwater G, et al. A multicenter prospective evaluation of the clinical utility of F-18 FDG-PET/CT in patients with AJCC stage IIIB or IIIC extremity melanoma. Ann Surg. 2012;256:350–6.
6. Carlino MS, Saunders CA, Haydu LE, et al. (18) F-labelled fluorodeoxyglucose-positron emission tomography (FDG-PET) heterogeneity of response is prognostic in dabrafenib treated BRAF mutant metastatic melanoma. Eur J Cancer. 2013;49:395–402.
7. Bronstein Y, Ng CS, Hwu P, Hwu WJ. Radiologic manifestations of immune-related adverse events in patients with metastatic melanoma undergoing anti- CTLA-4 antibody therapy. AJR. 2011;197:W992–W1000.
8. Perng P, Marcus C, Subramaniam RM. (18)F-FDG PET/CT and melanoma: staging, immune modulation and mutation-targeted therapy assessment, and prognosis. AJR Am J Roentgenol. 2015;205:259–70.
9. Rohren EM. PET/computed tomography and patient outcomes in melanoma. PET Clin. 2015;10:243–54.
10. Vidal-Sicart S, Rubello D, Pons F. Recurrence of melanoma. PET Clin. 2011;6:55–70.
11. Corrigan AJ, Schleyer PJ, Cook GJ. Pitfalls and artifacts in the use of PET/CT in oncology imaging. Semin Nucl Med. 2015;45(6):481–99.
12. Fuster D, Pons F, Rubello D, Alavi A. Other PET tracers and prospects for the future. PET Clin. 2011;6(1):91–7.
13. Grassetto G, Fuster D, Alavi A, Rubello D. Ocular melanoma and other unusual sites. PET Clin. 2011;6(1):79–89.
14. Krug B, Crott R, Roch I, et al. Cost-effectiveness analysis of FDG PET-CT in the management of pulmonary metastases from malignant melanoma. Acta Oncol. 2010;49(2):192–200.

Hepatocellular Cancer

9

1. What are the common indications of ¹⁸F-fluorodeoxyglucose (18F-FDG) posi-tron emission tomography (PET)-computed tomography (CT) in hepatocellular carcinoma (HCC)?

    18F-FDG-PET/CT is not very useful in diagnosing HCC because of its low sensitivity, particularly in detecting low-grade HCC. However, it provides use-ful information about the prognosis. 18F-FDG-PET/CT is used in detecting metastases and recurrent disease [1].

2. What is the role of 18F-FDG PET in diagnosing HCC?

    18F-FDG PET is of limited value in diagnosing HCC due to its low sensitiv-ity, as FDG uptake is variable in HCC depending on tumor grade. However, 18F-FDG PET-CT offers valuable prognostic information as well as implica-tions on further management such as liver transplantation, resection, liver-directed treatments, or sorafenib therapy [2, 3].

3. What is the role of 18F-FDG PET in staging HCC cancer?

    18F-FDG-PET/CT is useful in detecting extrahepatic (lymph nodal and dis-tant) metastases and was found to be more accurate in detecting bone metasta-ses when compared to bone scan or CT [4–6].

4. What is the role of 18F-FDG PET in re-staging HCC?

    18F-FDG-PET/CT is useful in restaging of HCC with sensitivity and speci-ficity of 81.7% and 88.9%, respectively [4, 7].

5. What is the role of 18F-FDG PET in the assessment of treatment response in HCC?

    Early studies suggest that 18F-FDG PET/CT may play a role in the evalua-tion of treatment response after interventional loco-regional therapies for HCC and may perform better than morphological imaging, as they are insensitive in monitoring response, owing to the presence of necrosis, edema, hemorrhage, and cystic changes, when compared to metabolic imaging. However, further studies with many patients are needed to substantiate these results [8, 9].

© The Author(s), under exclusive license to Springer Nature
Switzerland AG 2026
S. Raja et al., *Question and Answers in PET/CT*,
https://doi.org/10.1007/978-3-032-00821-3_9

6. What are the sensitivity and specificity of 18F-FDG PET/CT in the assessment of distant metastasis?

A recent systematic review and meta-analysis demonstrated pooled sensitivity and specificity of 18F-FDG PET/CT for detecting metastatic HCC at 76.6% and 98.0%, respectively [4].

7. What is the role of 18F-FDG PET-CT in T staging?

18F-FDG PET has limited value in the T staging of HCC due to its low sensitivity and limited spatial resolution. Multi-phase CT and magnetic resonance imaging (MRI) are imaging modalities of choice for T staging of HCC [10, 11].

8. What is the role of 18F-FDG PET-CT in N staging?

18F-FDG PET/CT is useful in detecting lymph node metastasis in HCC patients with a sensitivity and specificity of 66.7% and 91.7%, respectively [5].

9. What is the role of 18F-FDG PET-CT in M staging?

18F-FDG PET/CT is useful in M staging of HCC with pooled sensitivity and specificity of 76.6% and 98%, respectively. It also performs better than CT or bone scintigraphy in detecting bone metastases [4, 5].

10. What are the common pitfalls of 18F-FDG PET-CT in HCC?

The most common pitfall of 18F-FDG PET-CT in HCC is variable FDG avidity based on the tumor grade, resulting in low sensitivity [3].

11. What are the common false-positive 18F-FDG PET-CT findings in HCC?

Common false-positive 18F-FDG PET-CT findings include infection/ inflammatory conditions such as liver abscess/cholangitis, physiological bowel/ urinary tracer activity, treatment-related changes like hematoma and post-radiotherapy inflammation, and so on. In addition, various artifacts related to misregistration, partial volume effect, attenuation correction, and truncation artifacts can result in false positives [1, 12].

12. What are the common false-negative 18F-FDG PET-CT findings in HCC?

Common false-negative 18F-FDG PET-CT findings in HCC are as follows:

(a) Low-grade/well-differentiated HCC
(b) Small-sized lesions/lymph nodes (smaller than the resolution of the PET scanner)
(c) Post-chemotherapy status
(d) Artifacts like misregistration artifact, and so on [1, 12]

13. What are the methods to improve the sensitivity of 18F-FDG PET/CT in detecting HCC?

Methods to improve the sensitivity of 18F-FDG PET/CT in detecting HCC are delayed imaging at 2 or 3 h after FDG administration and incorporation of early dynamic images following FDG administration by demonstrating higher arterial perfusion of HCC [13–15].

14. What are non-FDG tracers used in imaging HCC?

    Because of the higher false negative rate of 18F FDG PET/CT in detecting well-differentiated HCC, other tracers like 11C/18F labeled Acetate or Choline (Radiotracers of lipogenesis) have been explored, and their reported sensitivity is more than 85%. These tracers are complementary to 18F-FDG, and dual tracer imaging (18F-FDG and one of the lipogenesis radiotracers) seems to be more accurate and yield the most information for detecting and characterizing HCC [1, 16, 17]. If short-lived isotopes such as 11C are used, dual isotope imaging can be performed on the same day, using 11C acetate or choline first. In recent years, there have been proposals to use 68Ga-Prostate Specific Membrane Antigen (PSMA) to image the neovascularity in HCC, given the convenience of this generator-based tracer.

15. What is the role of 18F-FDG PET-CT in radiotherapy planning in HCC?

    18F-FDG PET-CT may be useful in selecting HCC patients who are likely to respond to radiotherapy, as few studies have shown that patients with high Standardised Uptake Value (SUV) ratios are more likely to show objective tumor response to radiotherapy than those with low SUV ratios [18, 19].

16. What are the advantages and limitations of 18F-FDG PET-CT in HCC?

    Advantages: 18F-FDG PET-CT is useful in detecting extrahepatic metastases and in the surveillance and prognostication of HCC. It may also have a role in the treatment response assessment of HCC following loco-regional therapies.

    Limitations: Since FDG uptake is variable in HCC depending on tumor grade, 18F-FDG PET/CT has low sensitivity in diagnosing well-differentiated HCC [1–3].

17. What is the role of 18F-FDG PET-CT in the management of cholangiocarcinoma?

    Morphologic characteristics and location of lesions influence the sensitivity of 18F-FDG PET/CT in the diagnosis of cholangiocarcinoma, which is higher (more than 85%) for nodular forms and peripherally located lesions and low (18–58%) for periductal infiltrating and hilar cholangiocarcinoma. However, 18F-FDG PET/CT is very beneficial in detecting lymph nodal (with the highest accuracy of 86%, compared to 68% and 57% for CT and MRI, respectively) and distant metastases from cholangiocarcinoma, which can affect patient management (up to 30%). It is also useful in treatment response assessment and detecting recurrence [20–22].

References

1. Jadvar H. Hepatocellular carcinoma and gastroenteropancreatic neuroendocrine tumors: potential role of other positron emission tomography radiotracers. Semin Nucl Med. 2012;42(4):247–54.
2. Sun DW, An L, Wei F, Mu L, Shi XJ, Wang CL, et al. Prognostic significance of parameters from pretreatment (18)F-FDG PET in hepatocellular carcinoma: a meta-analysis. Abdom Radiol (NY). 2016;41:33–41.

3. Haug AR. Imaging of primary liver tumors with positron-emission tomography. Q J Nucl Med Mol Imaging. 2017;61(3):292–300.
4. Lin CY, Chen JH, Liang JA, Lin CC, Jeng LB, Kao CH. 18F-FDG PET or PET/CT for detecting extrahepatic metastases or recurrent hepatocellular carcinoma: a systematic review and meta-analysis. Eur J Radiol. 2012;81(9):2417–22.
5. Kawaoka T, Aikata H, Takaki S, et al. FDG positronemission tomography/computed tomography for the detection of extrahepatic metastases from hepatocellular carcinoma. Hepatol Res. 2009;39(2):134–42.
6. Lee JE, Jang JY, Jeong SW, et al. Diagnostic value for extrahepatic metastases of hepatocellular carcinoma in positron emission tomography/computed tomography scan. World J Gastroenterol. 2012;18(23):2979–87.
7. Han A, Gwak G, Choi M, et al. The clinical value of 18F-FDG-PET/CT for investigating unexplained serum AFP elevation following interventional therapy for hepatocellular carcinoma. Hepato Gastroenterol. 2009;56:1111–6.
8. Kim SH, Won KS, Choi BW, et al. Usefulness of F-18 FDG PET/CT in the evaluation of early treatment response after interventional therapy for hepatocellular carcinoma. Nucl Med Mol Imaging. 2012;46(2):102–10.
9. Dierckx R, Maes A, Peeters M, Van De Wiele C. FDG PET for monitoring response to local and locoregional therapy in HCC and liver metastases. Q J Nucl Med Mol Imaging. 2009;53(3):336–42.
10. European Association for the Study of the Liver, European Organisation for Research, Treatment of Cancer. EASL-EORTC clinical practice guidelines: management of hepatocellular carcinoma. J Hepatol. 2012;56:908–43.
11. Bruix J, Sherman M, American Association for the Study of Liver Diseases. Management of hepatocellular carcinoma: an update. Hepatology. 2011;53:1020–2.
12. Corrigan AJ, Schleyer PJ, Cook GJ. Pitfalls and artifacts in the use of PET/CT in oncology imaging. Semin Nucl Med. 2015;45(6):481–99.
13. Bernstine H, Braun M, Yefremov N, et al. FDG-PET/CT early dynamic blood flow and late standardized uptake value determination in hepatocellular carcinoma. Radiology. 2011;260:503–10.
14. Wang SB, Wu HB, Wang QS, Zhou WL, Tian Y, Li HS, et al. Combined early dynamic (18) F-FDG PET/CT and conventional whole-body (18)F-FDG PET/CT provide one-stop imaging for detecting hepatocellular carcinoma. Clin Res Hepatol Gastroenterol. 2015;39:324–30.
15. Wu B, Zhao Y, Zhang Y, Tan H, Shi H. Does dual-time-point 18F-FDG PET/CT scan add in the diagnosis of hepatocellular carcinoma? Hell J Nucl Med. 2017;20(1):79–82.
16. Ho CL, Yu SC, Yeung DW. 11C-acetate PET imaging in hepatocellular carcinoma and other liver masses. J Nucl Med. 2003;44:213–21.
17. Talbot JN, Fartoux L, Balogova S. Detection of hepatocellular carcinoma with PET/CT: a prospective comparison of 18F-Fluorocholine and 18F-FDG in patients with cirrhosis or chronic liver disease. J Nucl Med. 2010;51:1699–706.
18. Kim JW, Seong J, Yun M, et al. Usefulness of positron emission tomography with Fluorine-18-Fluorodeoxyglucose in predicting treatment response in Unresectable hepatocellular carcinoma patients treated with external beam radiotherapy. Int J Radiat Oncol Biol Phys. 2012;82(3):1172–8.
19. In Young Jo, Seok-Hyun Son, Myungsoo Kim, et al. Prognostic value of pretreatment 18F-FDG PET-CT in radiotherapy for patients with hepatocellular carcinoma. Radiat Oncol J. 2015;33(3):179–87.
20. Sacks A, Peller PJ, Surasi DS, Chatburn L, Mercier G, Subramaniam RM. Value of PET/CT in the management of primary hepatobiliary tumors, part 2. AJR Am J Roentgenol. 2011;197(2):W260–5.
21. Seo S, Hatano E, Higashi T, et al. Fluorine-18 fluorodeoxyglucose positron emission tomography predicts lymph node metastasis, P-glycoprotein expression, and recurrence after resection in mass-forming intrahepatic cholangiocarcinoma. Surgery. 2008;143:769–77.
22. Park TG, Schmidt F, Caca K, et al. Implication of lymph node metastasis detected on 18F-FDG PET/ CT for surgical planning in patients with peripheral intrahepatic cholangiocarcinoma. Clin Nucl Med. 2014;39(1):1–7.

1. What are the common indications of ^{18}F-fluorodeoxyglucose (18F-FDG) positron emission tomography (PET)-computed tomography (CT) in gall bladder cancer?

   The common indications of 18F-FDG PET-CT in gall bladder cancer are as follows:

   (a) Evaluation of suspicious gall bladder lesions for diagnosis
   (b) Assessment of distant metastases
   (c) Evaluation of suspected recurrence
   (d) Prognostication [1, 2]

2. What is the role of 18F-FDG PET-CT in diagnosing gall bladder cancer?

   18F-FDG PET-CT is useful in the diagnosis of gall bladder cancer with an overall accuracy of more than 95% [1–3].

3. What is the role of 18F-FDG PET-CT in staging gall bladder cancer?

   Initial studies show that 18F-FDG PET-CT is useful and superior to conventional imaging in detecting distant metastases in gall bladder cancer with an accuracy of more than 95%. However, the accuracy of 18F-FDG PET-CT is relatively low (approximately 85%) for detecting lymph nodal metastases. T staging can be done accurately if the PET/CT protocol includes contrast-enhanced CT. However, further validation in large prospective studies is required [1, 2].

4. What is the role of 18F-FDG PET-CT in re-staging gall bladder cancer?

   After cholecystectomy, incidental gallbladder cancer requires an accurate staging method to identify residual or metastatic disease and determine resectability. Initial studies show that 18F-FDG PET/CT is more precise (accuracy ranging from 90% to 100%) in this clinical setting and helpful primarily in

S. Raja et al., *Question and Answers in PET/CT*,
https://doi.org/10.1007/978-3-032-00821-3_10

avoiding surgical exploration for those with unresectable and/or disseminated disease. 18F-FDG PET/CT is also more accurate in detecting tumor recurrence during follow-up, with a sensitivity of 97.6% and specificity of 90%. These findings need further validation in large prospective studies [4–7].

5. What is the role of 18F-FDG PET-CT in the assessment of treatment response in gall bladder cancer?

    Although initial studies show 18F-FDG PET-CT in the assessment of treatment response in gall bladder cancer, particularly in those patients where metallic artifacts from the cholecystectomy surgical clips or a biliary stent distort findings, this needs further validation in large prospective studies [8].

6. What are the sensitivity and specificity of 18F-FDG PET-CT in the assessment of distant metastasis of gall bladder cancer?

    Initial studies show a sensitivity of up to 100% and more than 90% specificity for 18F-FDG PET-CT in detecting distant metastases from gall bladder cancer [2, 9].

7. What is the role of 18F-FDG PET-CT in T staging?

    The role of 18F-FDG PET-CT is limited in staging gall bladder cancer. However, if contrast-enhanced CT is included in the PET/CT protocol, it gives accurate information about T staging of gall bladder cancer [1].

8. What is the role of 18F-FDG PET-CT in N staging?

    Even though 18F-FDG PET-CT is more specific (usually more than 95%) in detecting lymph nodal metastases in gall bladder cancer, its sensitivity is low (approximately 60–70%), mainly due to its inability to detect small metastatic lymph nodes as well as interference by strong photon scatter from an avidly hypermetabolic primary mass [1, 2].

9. What is the role of 18F-FDG PET-CT in M staging?

    18F-FDG PET-CT is useful in detecting distant metastases with an accuracy of more than 95% [1, 2].

10. What are the common pitfalls of 18F-FDG PET-CT in gall bladder cancer?

    The common pitfalls of 18F-FDG PET-CT in gall bladder cancer include various inflammatory conditions like acute/xanthogranulomatous cholecystitis, which may mimic gall bladder cancer. 18F-FDG PET CT may also be negative in a mucinous variant of gall bladder cancer. Only a limited number of studies are available regarding the role of 18F-FDG PET CT in gall bladder cancer. Larger prospective studies are needed to validate its role [1–3].

11. What are the common false-positive 18F-FDG PET-CT findings in gall bladder cancer?

    The common false-positive 18F-FDG PET-CT findings in pancreatic cancer are as follows:

    (a) Any   infection/inflammation   (e.g.,   acute/xantho   granulomatous cholecystitis).

(b) Increased metabolic activity in Rokwitansky–Aschoff sinus or adenomyomatosis.

(c) Physiological accumulation of 18F-FDG within the gallbladder vesicle due to excretion.

(d) Treatment-induced inflammatory changes following radiotherapy, recent surgery, and so on.

(e) Physiological bowel/urinary tracer activity.

(f) Various artifacts such as misregistration artifact, partial volume effect, attenuation correction artifact, truncation artifact, and so on [10–14]

12. What are the common false-negative 18F-FDG PET-CT findings in gall bladder cancer?

   Common false-negative 18F-FDG PET-CT findings are as follows:

(a) Mucinous/necrotic tumors.

(b) Small-sized lesions/lymph nodes (smaller than the resolution of the PET scanner),

(c) Post-chemotherapy status.

(d) Artifacts like misregistration artifacts [1, 2, 14]

13. What is the role of 18F-FDG PET-CT in radiotherapy planning in gall bladder cancer?

   The role of 18F-FDG PET-CT in radiotherapy planning in gall bladder cancer has not been studied adequately.

14. What are the advantages and limitations of 18F-FDG PET-CT in gall bladder cancer?

   Advantages: 18F-FDG PET/CT is highly accurate in detecting gall bladder cancer and distant metastases and disease recurrence during follow-up. It is also helpful in prognostication.

   Limitations: The accuracy of 18F-FDG PET/CT in detecting lymph nodal metastases is relatively low, and its role in treatment response assessment is not well known. Overall, only a limited number of studies are available regarding the role of 18F-FDG PET-CT in gall bladder cancer. Larger prospective studies are needed to validate its role [1, 2, 7, 15, 16].

References

1. Parikh U, Marcus C, Sarangi R, Taghipour M, Subramaniam RM. FDG PET/CT in Pancreatic and Hepatobiliary Carcinomas: Value to Patient Management and Patient Outcomes. PET Clin. 2015;10(3):327–43.
2. Ramos-Font C, Gómez-Rio M, Rodríguez-Fernández A, Jiménez-Heffernan A, Sánchez Sánchez R, Llamas-Elvira JM. Ability of FDG-PET/CT in the detection of gallbladder cancer. J Surg Oncol. 2014;109(3):218–24.
3. Annunziata S, Pizzuto DA, Caldarella C, Galiandro F, Sadeghi R, Treglia G. Diagnostic accuracy of fluorine-18-fluorodeoxy glucose positron emission tomography in gallbladder cancer: A meta-analysis. World J Gastroenterol. 2015;21(40):11481–8.

 4. Kula Z, Malkowski B, Pietrzak T, et al. Initial evaluation of PET/CT imaging in patients with gallbladder carcinoma detected incidentally during or after cholecystectomy. Nowotwory. 2007;57:225e–9e.
 5. Shukla PJ, Barreto SG, Arya S, et al. Does PET-CT scan have a role prior to radical re-resection for incidental gallbladder cancer? HPB (Oxford). 2008;10:439–45.
 6. Butte JM, Redondo F, Waugh E, et al. The role of PET-CT in patients with incidental gallbladder cancer. HPB (Oxford). 2009;11:585–91.
 7. Kumar R, Sharma P, Kumari A, Halanaik D, Malhotra A. Role of 18F-FDG PET/CT in detecting recurrent gallbladder carcinoma. Clin Nucl Med. 2012;37(5):431–5.
 8. Shaikh F, Awan O, Khan SA. 18F-FDG PET/CT Imaging of Gall bladder Adenocarcinoma—A Pictorial Review. Cureus. 2015;7(8):e298.
 9. Lee SW, Kim HJ, Park JH, et al. Clinical usefulness of 18F-FDG PET-CT for patients with gallbladder cancer and cholangiocarcinoma. J Gastroenterol. 2010;45(5):560–6.
10. Rodríguez-Fernández A, Gómez-Río M, Llamas-Elvira JM, et al. Positron-emission tomography with fluorine-18- fluoro-2- deoxy-Dglucose for gallbladder cancer diagnosis. Am J Surg. 2004;188:171–5.
11. Rodríguez-Fernández A, Gómez-Río M, Llamas-Elvira JM. Functional imaging. In: Thomas CR, Fuller CD, editors. Billiary tract and gallbladder cancer. New York: Demos Medical Publishing; 2009. p. 131–9.
12. Maldjian PD, Ghesani N, Ahned S, et al. Adenomyomatosis of the gallbladder: another cause for a "hot" gallbladder on 18F-FDG PET. AJR Am J Roentgenol. 2007;189:W36–8.
13. Murata Y, Watanabe H, Kubota K, et al. PET/CT evaluation of the physiologic accumulation of 18F-FDG within the gallbladder vesicle. Nucl Med Biol. 2007;34:961–6.
14. Corrigan AJ, Schleyer PJ, Cook GJ. Pitfalls and artifacts in the use of PET/CT in oncology imaging. Semin Nucl Med. 2015;45(6):481–99.
15. Redondo F, Butte J, Lavados H, et al. 18F-FDG PET/CT performance and prognostic value in patients with incidental gallbladder carcinoma. J Nucl Med. 2012;53(515):515.
16. Hwang JP, Lim I, Na II, et al. Prognostic value of SUV Max measured by fluorine-18 fluorodeoxyglucose positron emission tomography with computed tomography in patients with gallbladder cancer. Nucl Med Mol Imaging. 2014;48(2):114–20.

1. What are the common indications of ^{18}F-fluorodeoxyglucose (18F-FDG) positron emission tomography (PET)-computed tomography (CT) in pancreatic cancer?

    The common indications of 18F-FDG PET-CT in pancreatic cancer are as follows:

    (a) Assessment of distant metastasis
    (b) Monitoring treatment response
    (c) Detection of suspected recurrence
    (d) Guiding the site of tissue sampling for diagnosis [1–3]

2. What is the role of 18F-FDG PET-CT in diagnosing pancreatic cancer?

    Even though 18F-FDG PET-CT is highly sensitive in the diagnosis of pancreatic cancer (with a sensitivity of more than 85%), the specificity is relatively low (ranging from 50% to 87%), mainly because of its inability to accurately differentiate pancreatic cancer from mass-forming pancreatitis [2, 4–6].

3. What are the typical findings of 18F-FDG PET-CT in the evaluation of pancreatic diseases?

    One key differentiating feature between pancreatic carcinoma and pancreatitis is the distribution of 18F-FDG uptake. Focal uptake tends to be seen in pancreatic cancer, and diffuse uptake is usually found in pancreatitis (the exception being mass-forming pancreatitis). If diffuse pancreatic uptake is associated with increased salivary gland uptake, it is more indicative of autoimmune pancreatitis [3, 7].

4. What is the role of 18F-FDG PET-CT in staging pancreatic cancer?

    18F-FDG PET-CT is not very useful in the assessment of the primary site (CECT is the modality of choice for assessing resectability), as well as lymph nodal metastases (even though 18F-FDG PET-CT is relatively more specific, sensitivity is very low). However, it is useful in detecting distant metastases and may change the management in up to 25–30% of patients [2, 3, 8].

5. What is the role of 18F-FDG PET-CT in re-staging pancreatic cancer?

   18F-FDG PET-CT is useful in restaging treated pancreatic cancer patients with rising CA-19-9 levels, as it detects the relapse much earlier than CT [1, 2, 9].

6. What is the role of 18F-FDG PET-CT in the assessment of treatment response in pancreatic cancer?

   18F-FDG PET-CT seems to be a more effective method for evaluating tumor response than conventional CT following radiotherapy or chemotherapy for unresectable pancreatic cancer because of its ability to detect the metabolic change before the morphological changes. However, this needs to be validated in larger prospective studies [10, 11].

7. What is the role of 18F-FDG PET-CT in T staging?

   18F-FDG PET with non-contrast CT is of very little value in T staging of pancreatic cancer. However, 18F-FDG PET with contrast-enhanced CT is accurate in T staging, particularly in assessing local tumor invasion and involvement of major vascular structures, which is the most critical factor for resectability [12].

8. What is the role of 18F-FDG PET-CT in N staging?

   Despite its relatively high specificity (63–93%), 18F-FDG PET-CT has low sensitivity (30–50%) in detecting lymph nodal metastases from pancreatic cancer, mainly due to its inability to detect small metastatic lymph nodes as well as interference by strong photon scatter from an avidly hypermetabolic primary mass [8, 13].

9. What is the role of 18F-FDG PET-CT in M staging?

   18F-FDG PET-CT is useful in detecting metastases from pancreatic cancer. The accuracy of 18F-FDG PET-CT is higher than conventional imaging in detecting distant metastases, particularly in bones and lungs. However, MRI is relatively more accurate in identifying liver metastases, particularly smaller ones. This may be due to its limited spatial resolution, partial volume effect, high metabolic background of the liver, and so on. Pancreatic adenocarcinoma tends to metastasize to the peritoneum, rendering patients ineligible for surgery. Even though 18F-FDG PET-CT performs better than CT, all the imaging modalities have limited accuracy in identifying smaller peritoneal deposits compared to staging laparoscopy/laparotomy [2, 13–16].

10. What are the common pitfalls of 18F-FDG PET-CT in pancreatic cancer?

   The accuracy of 18F-FDG PET-CT in assessing local invasion and regional lymph nodal metastases is not optimal. However, including CECT in the PET-CT protocol may improve the accuracy. Its sensitivity is also limited in mucinous (due to tissue hypocellularity), necrotic tumors, and liver and peritoneal metastases smaller than 1 cm. Its value in the treatment response assessment and prognostication is yet to be proven [2, 13].

11. What are the common false-positive 18F-FDG PET-CT findings in pancreatic cancer?

The common false-positive 18F-FDG PET-CT findings in pancreatic cancer are as follows:

(a) Any infection/inflammation (e.g., mass-forming pancreatitis, tuberculosis, acute/chronic pancreatitis, etc.)
(b) Treatment-induced inflammatory changes following radiotherapy, recent surgery/biopsy, CBD stenting, etc.
(c) Physiological bowel/urinary tracer activity
(d) Various artifacts like misregistration artifact, partial volume effect, attenuation correction artifact, truncation artifact, and so on [2, 13, 17]

12. What are the common false-negative 18F-FDG PET-CT findings in pancreatic cancer?

The common false-negative 18F-FDG PET-CT findings in pancreatic cancer are as follows:

(a) Mucinous/necrotic tumors
(b) Small-sized (mainly primary, liver and peritoneal) lesions/lymph nodes (smaller than the resolution of the PET scanner)
(c) Post-chemotherapy status
(d) Misregistration artifacts [2, 13, 17]

13. What are non-FDG tracers in imaging pancreatic cancer?

Because of its higher specificity for tumor cells, 18F-fluorothymidine (FLT—a proliferation marker) is being evaluated in pancreatic cancer, and its role is yet to be validated. The major disadvantage is its poor sensitivity in detecting liver metastases due to high physiological FLT liver uptake.

(a) Hypoxia tracers like 18F-Fluoromisonidazole (FMISO) are also being evaluated
(b) Other tracers being used in the evaluation of neuroendocrine tumors of the pancreas include gallium-68-labeled somatostatin analogs (^{68}Ga-DOTA-d-Phe1-Tyr3-octreotide (DOTATOC), ^{68}Ga-DOTA-Tyr3-octreotate (DOTATATE), and ^{68}Ga-DOTA-1-Nal3-octreotide (DOTANOC))
(c) ^{18}F-fluorodihydroxyphenylalanine
(d) ^{68}Ga NOTA-exendin-4
(e) ^{124}I-metaiodobenzylguanidine
(f) β-[^{11}C]-5-hydroxy-L-tryptophan
(g) Gallium-68 fibroblast activated protein [18–22]

14. What is the role of 18F-FDG PET-CT in radiotherapy planning in pancreatic cancer?

The local recurrence rate following chemoradiation in unresectable locally advanced pancreatic cancer is around 42–68%, which is exceptionally high and may be due to geographic misses. Recent studies show that 18F-FDG PET/CT increases the extent of gross tumor volume and planning target volume in up to 35% of patients. This would avoid geographic misses and deliver more radiation dose to the tumor, thereby reducing the recurrence rate. However, this needs to be validated in larger prospective studies [13, 23]

15. What is the cost-effectiveness of 18F-FDG PET-CT pancreatic cancer?

A few studies have shown that 18F-FDG PET-CT detects additional distant metastases/synchronous second primary malignancies in many patients and changes the management, thereby reducing the cost. However, this needs to be validated in larger prospective studies [24, 25]

16. What are the advantages and limitations of 18F-FDG PET-CT in pancreatic cancer?

Advantages: 18F-FDG PET-CT is useful in assessing distant metastasis or suspected recurrence and guiding the site of tissue sampling for diagnosis.

Limitations: The accuracy of 18F-FDG PET-CT in assessing local invasion and regional lymph nodal metastases is not optimal (which could be overcome by incorporating CECT in the PET-CT protocol). Its sensitivity is also limited in mucinous (due to tissue hypocellularity) and necrotic tumors, as well as in detecting small liver and peritoneal metastases. Its value in the treatment response assessment and prognostication is yet to be proven.

References

1. Sahani DV, Bonaffini PA, Catalano OA, Guimaraes AR, Blake MA. State-of-the-art PET/CT of the pancreas: current role and emerging indications. Radiographics. 2012;32(4):1133–58.
2. Wang XY, Yang F, Jin C, Fu DL. Utility of PET/CT in diagnosis, staging, assessment of resectability and metabolic response of pancreatic cancer. World J Gastroenterol. 2014;20(42):15580–9.
3. Parikh U, Marcus C, Sarangi R, Taghipour M, Subramaniam RM. FDG PET/CT in pancreatic and hepatobiliary carcinomas: value to patient management and patient outcomes. PET Clin. 2015;10(3):327–43.
4. Tang S, Huang G, Liu J, Liu T, Treven L, Song S, Zhang C, Pan L, Zhang T. Usefulness of 18F-FDG PET, combined FDG-PET/CT and EUS in diagnosing primary pancreatic carcinoma: a meta-analysis. Eur J Radiol. 2011;78:142–50.
5. Wu LM, Hu JN, Hua J, Liu MJ, Chen J, Xu JR. Diagnostic value of diffusion-weighted magnetic resonance imaging compared with fluorodeoxyglucose positron emission tomography/computed tomography for pancreatic malignancy: a meta-analysis using a hierarchical regression model. J Gastroenterol Hepatol. 2012;27:1027–35.
6. Rijkers AP, Valkema R, Duivenvoorden HJ, et al. Usefulness of F-18-fluorodeoxyglucose positron emission tomography to confirm suspected pancreatic cancer: a meta-analysis. Eur J Surg Oncol. 2014;40(7):794–804.
7. Lee TY, Kim MH, Park do H, et al. Utility of 18F-FDG PET/CT for differentiation of autoimmune pancreatitis with atypical pancreatic imaging findings from pancreatic cancer. AJR Am J Roentgenol. 2009;193(2):343–8.
8. Kauhanen SP, Komar G, Seppänen MP, et al. A prospective diagnostic accuracy study of 18F-fluorodeoxyglucose positron emission tomography/computed tomography, multidetector row computed tomography, and magnetic resonance imaging in primary diagnosis and staging of pancreatic cancer. Ann Surg. 2009;250(6):957–63.

9. Sperti C, Pasquali C, Bissoli S, Chierichetti F, Liessi G, Pedrazzoli S. Tumor relapse after pancreatic cancer resection is detected earlier by 18-FDG PET than by CT. J Gastrointest Surg. 2010;14:131–40.

10. Toesca DA, Pollom EL, Poullos PD, et al. Assessing local progression after stereotactic body radiation therapy for unresectable pancreatic adenocarcinoma: CT versus PET. Pract Radiat Oncol. 2017;7(2):120–5.

11. Kittaka H, Takahashi H, Ohigashi H, et al. Role of (18)F-fluorodeoxyglucose positron emission tomography/computed tomography in predicting the pathologic response to preoperative chemoradiation therapy in patients with resectable T3 pancreatic cancer. World J Surg. 2013;37(1):169–78.

12. Strobel K, Heinrich S, Bhure U, et al. Contrast-enhanced 18FFDG PET/CT: 1-stop-shop imaging for assessing the resectability of pancreatic cancer. J Nucl Med. 2008;49:1408–13.

13. Jha P, Bijan B. PET/CT for pancreatic malignancy: potential and pitfalls. J Nucl Med Technol. 2015;43(2):92–7.

14. Sahani DV, Kalva SP, Fischman AJ, et al. Detection of liver metastases from adenocarcinoma of the colon and pancreas: comparison of mangafodipir trisodium-enhanced liver MRI and whole-body FDG PET. AJR Am J Roentgenol. 2005;185(1):239–46.

15. Farma JM, Santillan AA, Melis M, Walters J, Belinc D, Chen DT, Eikman EA, Malafa M. PET/CT fusion scan enhances CT staging in patients with pancreatic neoplasms. Ann Surg Oncol. 2008;15:2465–71.

16. Liu RC, Traverso LW. Diagnostic laparoscopy improves staging of pancreatic cancer deemed locally unresectable by computed tomography. Surg Endosc. 2005;19(5):638–42.

17. Corrigan AJ, Schleyer PJ, Cook GJ. Pitfalls and artifacts in the use of PET/CT in oncology imaging. Semin Nucl Med. 2015;45(6):481–99.

18. Vineeth Kumar PM, Verma GR, Mittal BR, et al. FLT PET/CT is better than FDG PET/CT in differentiating benign from malignant pancreato biliary lesions. Clin Nucl Med. 2016;41(5):e244–50.

19. Nakajo M, Kajiya Y, Tani A, et al. A pilot study of the diagnostic and prognostic values of FLT-PET/CT for pancreatic cancer: comparison with FDG-PET/CT. Abdom Radiol (NY). 2017;42(4):1210–21.

20. Segard T, Robins PD, Yusoff IF, Ee H, Morandeau L, Campbell EM, Francis RJ. Detection of hypoxia with 18F-fluoromisonidazole (18F-FMISO) PET/CT in suspected or proven pancreatic cancer. Clin Nucl Med. 2013;38:1–6.

21. Koopmans KP, Glaudemans AW. Other PET tracers for neuroendocrine tumors. PET Clin. 2014;9:57–62.

22. Luo Y, Pan Q, Yao S, et al. Glucagon-like Peptide-1 receptor PET/CT with 68Ga-NOTA-exendin-4 for detecting localized insulinoma: a prospective cohort study. J Nucl Med. 2016;57:715–20.

23. Topkan E, Yavuz AA, Aydin M, et al. Comparison of CT and PET-CT based planning of radiation therapy in locally advanced pancreatic carcinoma. J Exp Clin Cancer Res. 2008;27:41–7.

24. Heinrich S, Goerres GW, Schafer M, et al. Positron emission tomography/computed tomography influences on the management of respectable pancreatic cancer and its cost-effectiveness. Ann Surg. 2005;242:235–43.

25. Dibble EH, Karantanis D, Mercier G, Peller PJ, Kachnic LA, Subramaniam RM. PET/CT of cancer patients: part 1, pancreatic neoplasms. AJR Am J Roentgenol. 2012;199(5):952–67.

Cholangiocarcinoma

1. What is cholangiocarcinoma?

   Cholangiocarcinoma (CCA), the second most common primary hepatic cancer, is a cancer of the bile duct. Based on its anatomical location, cholangiocarcinoma can be broadly classified as intrahepatic (5–10%) or extrahepatic. The extrahepatic cholangiocarcinoma is further classified as perihilar and distal (60–70% occur at the bifurcation of hepatic ducts, and 20–30% arise at the distal common bile) [1, 2]. Perihilar tumors, in turn, are further classified into four types according to the Bismuth–Corlette system, a significant tool in our understanding of cholangiocarcinoma [3].

2. What is the Bismuth–Corlette system classical of perihilar cholangiocarcinoma?

   Perihilar tumors are classified into four types based on the Bismuth–Corlette system [4]:

   Type 1—tumors below the confluence of the right and left hepatic ducts.

   Type 2—tumors reaching the confluence.

   Type 3—tumors involving the confluence and either the right (3a) or left (3b) hepatic ducts.

   Type 4—multicentric tumors or those involving the confluence and both the right and left ducts.

3. What is the classification of intrahepatic cholangiocarcinoma?

   Intrahepatic cholangiocarcinoma is divided into mass-forming, periductal, or intraductal based on the pattern of growth [3].

4. What are Klatskin tumors?

   The tumors that arise at the bifurcation site of the hepatic ducts (hilar) are called Klatskin tumors, which constitute 60–70% of the cholangiocarcinoma [1, 2].

S. Raja et al., *Question and Answers in PET/CT*, https://doi.org/10.1007/978-3-032-00821-3_12

5. What are the major risk factors for cholangiocarcinoma?

Primary sclerosing cholangitis and fibropolycystic liver disease (e.g., chole-dochal cysts) are the major risk factors for cholangiocarcinoma. Intrahepatic cholangiocarcinoma is reported to be associated with chronic liver disease and liver fluke infestation (e.g., chlonorchis sinensis). In addition, familial syndromes such as Lynch syndrome and biliary papillomatosis also predispose to cholangiocarcinoma [5].

6. What is the clinical manifestation of cholangiocarcinoma?

The extrahepatic cholangiocarcinoma presents with biliary tract obstruction. Intrahepatic cholangiocarcinoma is largely asymptomatic. Large intrahepatic masses may present with symptoms such as vague abdominal pain, anorexia, and weight loss [6].

7. What are the conventional imaging modalities used in imaging cholangiocarcinoma?

Ultrasound, computed tomography (CT), or magnetic resonance cholangiography are the common conventional imaging modalities used in imaging suspected cholangiocarcinoma. Endoscopic retrograde cholangiopancreatography helps in obtaining brush cytology and biopsy.

8. What are the common indications of ^{18}F-fluorodeoxyglucose (18F-FDG) positron emission tomography (PET)-CT in cholangiocarcinoma?

The common indications of 18F-FDG PET-CT in cholangiocarcinoma include the following:

(a) Diagnosis (suspected primary).
(b) Staging (primary staging and re-staging).
(c) Suspected recurrence.

9. What is the role of 18F-FDG PET-CT in diagnosing intrahepatic cholangiocarcinoma?

The sensitivity and specificity of 18F-FDG PET-CT are similar to CT or magnetic resonance imaging (MRI) for diagnosing satellite focus and vascular and bile duct invasion in patients with intrahepatic cholangiocarcinoma. However, 18F-FDG PET-CT is more accurate for diagnosing regional lymph node metastases. Overall, the accuracy of tumor staging by 18F-FDG PET-CT is relatively higher than that of CT or MRI [7].

10. What are the patterns of 18F-FDG uptake in cholangiocarcinoma?

Cholangiocarcinoma can show variable FDG uptake depending upon the anatomic location, growth pattern, and histological subtype [8–10].

11. What is the role of 18F-FDG PET-CT in detecting primary cholangiocarcinoma?

18F-FDG PET-CT has no clear advantage over these conventional imaging modalities in diagnosing cholangiocarcinoma. The accuracy of detection depends on the location of the lesion. Higher sensitivity and specificity are seen in detecting intrahepatic lesions, 91–95% and 80–100%, respectively [11–13]. The detection rate is also dependent on the patterns of growth.

12. What is the detection rate of 18F-FDG in mass-forming and infiltrative types of cholangiocarcinoma?

    The sensitivity for detection of a lesion is highest for mass-forming/nodular lesions compared to periductal or infiltrating lesions [9, 14–16]. The reported sensitivity is 85% for nodular lesions and 18% for infiltrative lesions [9, 16].

13. What is the role of 18F-FDG PET-CT in re-staging cholangiocarcinoma?

    18F-FDG PET-CT helps detect recurrent or metastatic disease, especially when other conventional imaging modalities are deemed inconclusive.

14. What is the sensitivity of FDG PET-CT in intra- and extrahepatic cholangiocarcinoma?

    1. Several studies indicate that the sensitivity of 18F-FDG PET-CT is higher in intrahepatic CCA than in perihilar and extrahepatic lesions. Corvera et al. showed that the sensitivity and specificity of 18F-FDG-PET in patients with suspected intrahepatic CCA are 95% and 100%, respectively, and in extrahepatic CCA, it is 69% and 67% [9].
    2. The detection rate of nodular tumors is higher than that of invasive tumors, and the sensitivity for nodular morphology is 85%, and for invasive morphology is 18% [12].

15. What are the sensitivity and specificity of 18F-FDG PET/CT in the diagnosis of the primary tumor?

    18F-FDG PET-CT in the diagnosis of the primary tumor showed a pooled sensitivity of 92% and a low pooled specificity of 51%, with the lowest specificity for hilar cholangiocarcinoma (22%) and extrahepatic cholangiocarcinoma (28%) [17].

16. What are the sensitivity and specificity of 18F-FDG PET/CT in the detection of lymph node metastases, distant metastases, and detection of relapse?

    1. Detection of lymph node metastases: Pooled sensitivity of 88% and specificity of 69%.
    2. Detection of distant metastases: Pooled sensitivity of 85% and specificity of 90%.
    3. Detection of relapse: Pooled sensitivity of 90% and specificity of 84% [17]

17. In what percentage of patients with cholangiocarcinoma does FDG PET-CT change the management?

    18F-FDG PET-CT changes the management in 15% of patients with cholangiocarcinoma [17].

18. In what percentage of patients does FDG PET-CT upstage the disease?

    18F-FDG PET-CT upstages the disease with the identification of previously unknown sites of disease in 78% of patients [17].

19. What is the role of 18F-FDG PET-CT in T staging of suspected and potentially operable cholangiocarcinoma?

    18F-FDG PET-CT is not superior to CT or MRI for assessing the primary tumors. However, it helps detect lymph nodes and distant metastases and helps in accurate staging.

20. What is the role of 18F-FDG PET-CT in N staging?

    FDG PET-CT shows significantly higher accuracy than CT in diagnosing regional lymph node metastases (76% vs. 61%). Seo et al. [18] also found FDG PET to be a more accurate and specific detector of lymph node metastases in 35 patients than CT or MRI. The diagnostic accuracies of FDG PET, CT, and MRI for the detection of lymph node metastasis were 86%, 68%, and 57%; the sensitivities were 43%, 43%, and 43%; and the specificities were 100%, 76%, and 64%, respectively.

21. What is the role of 18F-FDG PET-CT in M staging?

    PET-CT shows significantly higher accuracy than CT in diagnosing distant metastases (88% vs. 79%) [19].

22. What are the common false-positive 18F-FDG PET-CT findings in cholangiocarcinoma?

    The common causes of false-positive uptake include the following:

    1. Infection-related false positives within the bile duct, co-existence of biliary stents.
    2. Tuberculosis, adenomyomatosis, and cholecystitis.
    3. Langerhans cell histiocytosis, IgG4-related sclerosing cholangitis, adenomyomatosis, and Xanthogranulomatous cholecystitis (XGC) [20–27].

23 . What are the common false-negative 18F-FDG PET-CT findings in cholangiocarcinoma?

    False-negative 18F-FDG PET-CT findings in cholangiocarcinoma include small tumor size, low metabolic activity, and physiological liver activity, which can often mask subtle tumor uptake [2, 17].

24. What are non-FDG tracers in imaging cholangiocarcinoma?

    Cholangiocarcinoma is characterized by an intense desmoplastic reaction like that seen in pancreatic cancer. Several studies have reported FAPI-PET to have superior sensitivity than FDG-PET for primary cholangiocarcinoma (98% vs. 86%), lymph node metastases (90% vs. 87%), and distant metastases (100% vs. 84%) [28]. Higher tracer uptake was observed in FAPI-PET compared to FDG-PET for intrahepatic lesions, pelvic nodal metastases, and distant metastases, such as in the pleura or omentum. FAPI-PET led to changes in tumor staging in many patients [29, 30]. FAPI-PET demonstrates superior sensitivity to FDG-PET for cholangiocarcinoma, including at the disease's localized, locally advanced, and metastatic stages.

25. What is the role of 18F-FDG PET-CT in radiotherapy planning in cholangiocarcinoma?

    18F-FDG PET-CT is important in radiotherapy planning for cholangiocarcinoma. FDG PET-CT improves the accuracy of tumor delineation, guides treatment decisions, and optimizes radiation therapy.

26. What is the role of dual-time points ^{18}F-FDG PET-CT imaging in the primary diagnosis and staging of hilar cholangiocarcinoma?

    The delayed phase in dual time point 18F-FDG PET-CT scan is useful for detecting primary tumors and lymph node metastases in hilar cholangiocarcinoma. However, delayed PET-CT imaging did not benefit the detection of distant metastases. The sensitivity and accuracy of detection of primary lesions in the early phase were 69.6% and 70% versus 76.8% and 76.8% in the delay phase, respectively [31].

27. What are the advantages and limitations of 18F-FDG PET-CT in cholangiocarcinoma?

    Advantages include detecting small cholangiocarcinoma as well as lymph nodes and distant metastases.

    Limitations include extrahepatic cholangiocarcinoma and low-grade tumors that are challenging to detect because of reduced 18F-FDG or a high background signal.

References

1. Lee Y, Yoo IR, Boo SH, Kim H, Park HL, Hyun OJ. The role of F-18 FDG PET/CT in intrahepatic cholangiocarcinoma. Nucl Med Mol Imaging. 2017;51(1):69–78.
2. Sacks A, Peller PJ, Surasi DS, Chatburn L, Mercier G, Subramaniam RM. Value of PET/CT in the management of primary hepatobiliary tumors, part 2. AJR Am J Roentgenol. 2011;197(2):W260–5.
3. Blechacz BR, Gores GJ. Cholangiocarcinoma. Clin Liver Dis. 2008;12:131e50.
4. Bismuth H, Nakache R, Diamond T. Management strategies in resection for hilar cholangiocarcinoma. Ann Surg. 1992;215:31.
5. Lee SS, Kim MH, Lee SK, et al. Clinicopathologic review of 58 patients with biliary papillomatosis. Cancer. 2004;100:783.
6. Saha SK, Zhu AX, Fuchs CS, Brooks GA. Forty-year trends in cholangiocarcinoma incidence in the U.S.: intrahepatic disease on the rise. Oncologist. 2016;21:594.
7. Nishioka E, Tsurusaki M, Kozuki R, et al. Comparison of conventional imaging and 18F-fluorodeoxyglucose positron emission tomography/computed tomography in the diagnostic accuracy of staging in patients with intrahepatic cholangiocarcinoma. Diagnostics (Basel). 2022;12(11):2889.
8. Kato T, Tsukamoto E, Kuge Y, Katoh C, Nambu T, Nobuta A, et al. Clinical role of ^{18}F-FDG PET for initial staging of patients with extrahepatic bile duct cancer. Eur J Nucl Med. 2002;29:1047e54.
9. Anderson CD, Rice MH, Pinson CW, Chapman WC, Chari RS, Delbeke D. Fluorodeoxyglucose PET imaging in the evaluation of gallbladder carcinoma and cholangiocarcinoma. J Gastrointest Surg. 2004;8:90–7.

10. Fritscher-Ravens A, Bohuslavizki KH, Broering DC, Jenicke L, Schafer H, Buchert R, et al. FDG PET in the diagnosis of hilar cholangiocarcinoma. Nucl Med Commun. 2001;22:1277e85.
11. Moon CM, Bang S, Chung JB, Park SW, Song SY, Yun M, et al. Usefulness of 18F- fluorodeoxyglucose positron emission tomography in differential diagnosis and staging of cholangiocarcinomas. J Gastroenterol Hepatol. 2008;23:759e65.
12. Corvera CU, Blumgart LH, Akhurst T, DeMatteo RP, D'Angelica M, Fong Y, et al. 18F-fluorodeoxyglucose positron emission tomography influences management decisions in patients with biliary cancer. J Am Coll Surg. 2008;206:57e65.
13. Keiding S, Hansen SB, Rasmussen HH, Gee A, Kruse A, Roelsgaard K, et al. Detection of cholangiocarcinoma in primary sclerosing cholangitis by positron emission tomography. Hepatology. 1998;28:700e6.
14. Kluge R, Schmidt F, Caca K, Barthel H, Hesse S, Georgi P, et al. Positron emission tomography with [18F]fluoro-2-deoxy-Dglucosefor diagnosis and staging of bile duct cancer. Hepatology. 2001;33:1029e35.
15. Nakeeb A, Pitt HA, Sohn TA, et al. Cholangiocarcinoma: a spectrum of intrahepatic, perihilar, and distal tumors. Ann Surg. 1996;224:463–73. discussion 473–475
16. Jadvar H, Henderson RW, Conti PS. [F-18]Fluorodeoxyglucose positron emission tomography and positron emission tomography: computed tomography in recurrent and metastatic cholangiocarcinoma. J Comput Assist Tomogr. 2007;31:223–8.
17. Lamarca A, Barriuso J, Chander A, McNamara MG, Hubner RA, ÓReilly D, et al. (18) F-fluorodeoxyglucose positron emission tomography ((18)FDG-PET) for patients with biliary tract cancer: systematic review and meta-analysis. J Hepatol. 2019;71:115–29.
18. Seo S, Hatano E, Higashi T, et al. Fluorine-18 fluorodeoxyglucose positron emission tomography predicts lymph node metastasis, P-glycoprotein expression, and recurrence after resection in mass-forming intrahepatic cholangiocarcinoma. Surgery. 2008;143:769–77.
19. Kim JY, Kim MH, Lee TY, Hwang CY, Kim JS, Yun SC, Lee SS, Seo DW, Lee SK. Clinical role of 18F-FDG PET-CT in suspected and potentially operable cholangiocarcinoma: a prospective study compared with conventional imaging. Am J Gastroenterol. 2008;103(5):1145–51.
20. Paudyal B, Oriuchi N, Paudyal P, Tsushima Y, Higuchi T, Miyakubo M, et al. Clinicopathological presentation of varying 18F-FDG uptake and expression of glucose transporter 1 and hexokinase II in cases of hepatocellular carcinoma and cholangiocellular carcinoma. Ann Nucl Med. 2008;22:83–6.
21. Goel S, Aggarwal A, Iqbal A, Gupta M, Rao A, Singh S. 18-FDG PET-CT should be included in preoperative staging of gall bladder cancer. Eur J Surg Oncol. 2020;46:1711–6.
22. Maldjian PD, Ghesani N, Ahmed S, Liu Y. Adenomyomatosis of the gallbladder: another cause for a "hot" gallbladder on 18F-FDG PET. AJR Am J Roentgenol. 2007;189:W36–8.
23. Lee KF, Hung EH, Leung HH, Lai PB. A narrative review of gallbladder adenomyomatosis: what we need to know. Ann Transl Med. 2020;8:1600.
24. Zhao Z, Wang Y, Guan Z, Jin J, Huang F, Zhu J. Utility of FDG-PET/CT in the diagnosis of IgG4-related diseases. Clin Exp Rheumatol. 2016;34:119–25.
25. Jessop S, Crudgington D, London K, Kellie S, Howman Giles R. FDG PET-CT in pediatric langerhans cell histiocytosis. Pediatr Blood Cancer. 2020;67:e28034.
26. Jain S, Karunanithi S, Singla S, Kumar A, Bal C, Kumar R. ^{18}F-FDG PET/CT in worsening of primary sclerosing cholangitis concomitant with improved langerhans cell histiocytosis. Rev Esp Med Nucl Imagen Mol. 2014;33:386–7.
27. Prabhu M, Nisamudeen F, Vikas H. [18F]FDG PET/CT in benign and malignant diseases involving the biliary tract. Indian. J Nucl Med. 2024;39(3):185–90.

28. Jinghua L, et al. Clinical prospective study of Gallium 68 (68Ga)-labeled fibroblast-activation protein inhibitor PET/CT in the diagnosis of biliary tract carcinoma. Eur J Nucl Med Mol Imaging. 2023;50:2152–66.
29. Lan L, et al. Prospective comparison of 68Ga-FAPI versus 18F-FDG PET/CT for tumor staging in biliary tract cancers. Radiology. 2022;304:648–57.
30. Affo S, et al. Promotion of cholangiocarcinoma growth by diverse cancer-associated fibroblast subpopulations. Cancer Cell. 2021;39:866–882.e11.
31. Pang L, Bo X, Wang J, et al. Role of dual-time point 18F-FDG PET/CT imaging in the primary diagnosis and staging of hilar cholangiocarcinoma. Abdom Radiol. 2021;46:4138–47.

Renal Cell Carcinoma

13

1. What are the common types of renal cancers?

   Types of renal cancers include

   (a) Renal cell carcinoma (RCC) (clear cell (cc) variant—80%; papillary variant—10%; and chromophobe variant—5%)
   (b) Squamous cell
   (c) Sarcomatoid
   (d) Urothelial cancers
   (e) Leiomyosarcoma
   (f) Small-cell carcinomas
   (g) Neuroendocrine tumors
   (h) Lymphomas [1–3]

2. What is the role of ^{18}F-fluorodeoxyglucose (18F-FDG) positron emission tomography (PET)-computed tomography (CT) in renal cancer?

   18F-FDG PET/CT is being used in selected high-risk renal cancer patients for identifying distant metastases and characterization of potential tumor thrombus. In metastatic renal cancer, FDG PET/CT is also used to monitor targeted molecular therapies. It also gives information about prognosis and survival [2].

3. What is the role of 18F-FDG PET-CT in diagnosing renal cancer?

   Despite its high specificity (90%), 18F-FDG PET-CT is not very useful in primary RCC evaluation due to its low sensitivity (only approximately 60%). This is mainly because of many RCCs' lower metabolic status and the predominant renal excretion of 18F-FDG, making RCCs isointense with renal parenchyma, which is often difficult to differentiate. However, a few tumor subtypes, such as type II papillary and sarcomatoid cancers, are highly FDG avid [4, 5].

© The Author(s), under exclusive license to Springer Nature
Switzerland AG 2026
S. Raja et al., *Question and Answers in PET/CT*,
https://doi.org/10.1007/978-3-032-00821-3_13

4. What is the role of 18F-FDG PET-CT in staging of renal cancer?

In general, 18F-FDG PET-CT is not widely used to stage RCC. However, it may help determine whether a thrombus in the renal vein and inferior vena cava is malignant or bland. 18F-FDG PET-CT is also helpful in detecting extra renal (lymph nodal and distant) metastatic disease in high-risk RCCs [2, 6].

5. What is the role of 18F-FDG PET in re-staging renal cancer?

18F-FDG PET/CT can effectively be used for postoperative surveillance and restaging of high-risk RCC patients, especially when conventional imaging is not conclusive [7, 8].

6. What is the role of 18F-FDG PET in the assessment of treatment response in renal cancer?

Since metastatic RCC patients are treated with novel targeted therapies such as tyrosine kinase inhibitors, there is often little change in the size of these lesions, and some metastases even increase while the drug prolongs survival. Thus, response evaluation using structural imaging based on size criteria (RECIST) may not be appropriate, and 18F-FDG PET/CT is found to be more useful than RECIST criteria for the response evaluation of metastatic lesions, especially for skeletal lesions [2, 4, 9].

7. What are the sensitivity and specificity of 18F-FDG PET/CT in renal cancers?

The sensitivity and specificity of 18F-FDG PET/CT in identifying renal cancers are approximately 60% and 90%, respectively [4].

8. What are the sensitivity and specificity of 18F-FDG in the assessment of extra renal metastatic disease in renal cancer?

The pooled sensitivity and specificity of 18 F-FDG-PET/CT to detect extra-renal (loco-regional lymph nodal and distant) metastatic lesions are 91% and 88%, respectively [6].

9. What are the common pitfalls of 18F-FDG PET-CT in renal cancer?

18F-FDG PET-CT is not very useful in the evaluation of kidney lesions due to the lower metabolic status of many RCCs and due to physiological renal excretion of 18F-FDG, making RCCs isointense with renal parenchyma, which often becomes difficult to differentiate [2].

10. What are the common false-positive 18F-FDG PET-CT findings in renal cancer?

Common false-positive 18F-FDG PET-CT findings in renal cancer are physiological urinary tracer activity mimicking disease, active infection/inflammation, and treatment-related changes such as hematoma and chemotherapy-induced lung changes. In addition, various artifacts such as misregistration artifacts, partial volume effect, attenuation correction artifacts, and truncation artifacts can result in false positives and misregistration artifacts [2, 10].

11. What are the common false-negative 18F-FDG PET-CT findings in renal cancer?

Common false-negative 18F-FDG PET-CT findings in renal cancer are as follows:

(a) Low/variable FDG avidity of many RCC subtypes
(b) Small-sized lesions/lymph nodes (smaller than the resolution of the PET scanner)
(c) Artifacts like misregistration artifacts [2, 10]

12. What are non-FDG tracers used in imaging of renal cancer?

(a) 11C—acetate (absent or least renal excretion allows better evaluation of renal lesions)
(b) 18F-flouride (for assessment of skeletal lesions)
(c) 18F-flourothyomidine (FLT- proliferation marker)
(d) 68Ga-prostate-specific membrane antigen (PSMA)

The absence/nonfunctionality of the tumor suppressor protein, von Hippel–Lindau is the characteristic molecular finding of the ccRCC and resultant accumulation of hypoxia-inducible factors (HIF-1α and HIF-2α; acting as transcription factors) and overexpression of their transcriptional targets, such as vascular endothelial growth factor (VEGF), glucose transporters (Glut), hexokinase, and carbonic anhydrase IX (CA-IX) allows the development of following tracers for imaging ccRCCs.

(e) 8124I-cG250 (Girentuximab—monoclonal antibody to CA-IX)
(f) 89Zr-Bevacizumab (monoclonal antibody to VEGF-A)
(g) 18F-fluoromisonidazole (hypoxia marker) [3, 11]

13. What is the role of 124I-cG250 PET/CT in the evaluation of renal cancer?

Since more than 95% of ccRCCs express CA-IX on their cell membrane, 124I-cG250 PET/CT has a better sensitivity of 86% (when compared to 18F-FDG, which has a sensitivity of around 60%) with a specificity of 86% for detecting this subtype. 124I-cG250 PET/CT also provides prognostic information and predicts response to targeted therapy in ccRCC. However, it is negative in other renal cancer types (even in aggressive ones) and requires longer imaging time (3–7 days) due to slow clearance of the tracer [2, 3].

14. What is the role of 68Ga-PSMA PET/CT in the evaluation of renal cancer?

68Ga-PSMA PET/CT has been used in imaging of prostate cancer for the last few years. However, it has been noticed that PSMA, a type II integral membrane glycoprotein (a functional enzyme), is not specific to the prostate and has also been upregulated in the neovasculature of various solid tumors, including RCCs.

For ccRCC, the reported PSMA expression ranges from 80% to 100%, while in other carcinoma types such as chromophobe and papillary, the expression is not as common (30–60% and 0%, respectively). There is a limitation in using PSMA PET for detecting and characterizing primary renal tumors due to urinary excretion of 68Ga and PSMA expression in the kidney's proximal tubules. Initial studies show that 68Ga-PSMA PET may potentially have a role in the metastatic evaluation of advanced RCC, as it detected multiple additional lesions that were not evident on conventional imaging. Further studies are required to confirm these observations [12].

15. What are the advantages and limitations of 18F-FDG PET-CT in renal cancer?

Advantages: 18F-FDG PET/CT is being used in selected high-risk renal cancer patients for identifying distant metastases and if there is a potential tumor thrombus. In metastatic renal cancer, FDG PET/CT is also used to monitor targeted molecular therapies. It also gives information about prognosis and survival.

Limitations: 18F-FDG PET-CT is not very useful in the evaluation of primary kidney lesions due to the lower metabolic status of many RCCs and also due to the physiological renal excretion of 18F-FDG, making RCCs isointense with renal parenchyma, which often becomes difficult to differentiate [2, 3, 7].

References

1. Linehan WM, Vasselli J, Srinivasan R, et al. Genetic basis of cancer of the kidney: disease-specific approaches to therapy. Clin Cancer Res. 2004;10(18 Pt 2):6282S–9S.
2. Bouchelouche K, Choyke PL. PET/computed tomography in renal, bladder, and testicular cancer. PET Clin. 2015;10(3):361–74.
3. Khandani AH, Rathmell WK. Positron emission tomography in renal cell carcinoma: an imaging biomarker in development. Semin Nucl Med. 2012;42(4):221–30.
4. Caldarella C, Muoio B, Isgro MA, et al. The role of fluorine-18-fluorodeoxyglucose positron emission tomography in evaluating the response to tyrosinekinase inhibitors in patients with metastatic primary renal cell carcinoma. Radiol Oncol. 2014;48:219.
5. Makis W, Ciarallo A, Rakheja R, et al. Spectrum of malignant renal and urinary bladder tumors on 18F-FDG PET/CT: a pictorial essay. Clin Imaging. 2012;36:660.
6. Wang HY, Ding HJ, Chen JH, Chao CH, Lu YY, Lin WY, Kao CH. Meta-analysis of the diagnostic performance of [18F]FDG-PET and PET/CT in renal cell carcinoma. Cancer Imaging. 2012;12:464–74.
7. Liu Y. The place of FDG PET/CT in renal cell carcinoma: value and limitations. Front Oncol. 2016;6:201.
8. Smaldone MC, Uzzo RG. Balancing process and risk: standardizing post treatment surveillance for renal cell carcinoma. J Urol. 2013;190:417.
9. Farnebo J, Gryback P, Harmenberg U, et al. Volumetric FDG-PET predicts overall and progression free survival after 14 days of targeted therapy in metastatic renal cell carcinoma. BMC Cancer. 2014;14:408.
10. Corrigan AJ, Schleyer PJ, Cook GJ. Pitfalls and artifacts in the use of PET/CT in oncology imaging. Semin Nucl Med. 2015;45(6):481–99.

11. Van Es SC, Brouwers AH, Mahesh SVK, et al. 89Zr-bevacizumab PET: potential early indicator of Everolimus efficacy in patients with metastatic renal cell carcinoma. J Nucl Med. 2017;58(6):905–10.
12. Rhee H, Blazak J, Tham CM. Pilot study: use of gallium-68 PSMA PET for detection of metastatic lesions in patients with renal tumour. EJNMMI Res. 2016;6(1):76.

Urinary Bladder Cancer

14

1. What are the types of urinary bladder cancer?
   (a) Urothelial or transitional cell carcinoma (>90%)
   (b) Squamous cell carcinoma
   (c) Adenocarcinoma
   (d) Sarcoma
   (e) Small cell carcinoma (very rare but aggressive poorly differentiated neuro-endocrine epithelial bladder tumor)
   (f) Paraganglioma [1, 2]

2. What is the role of ^{18}F-fluorodeoxyglucose (18F-FDG) positron emission tomography (PET)-computed tomography (CT) in bladder cancer?
   The role of 18-FDG PET-CT is limited to evaluating superficial bladder tumors. Still, it helps stage and restage muscle-invasive bladder cancer, and it may also add significant prognostic information.

3. What is the role of 18F-FDG PET-CT in diagnosing bladder cancer?
   Cystoscopy and CT urography are the primary diagnostic tests for bladder cancer. Even though 18F-FDG PET-CT is reasonably accurate in detecting urinary bladder cancer compared to CT or magnetic resonance imaging (MRI), no superiority has been demonstrated over these conventional techniques in the evaluation of primary bladder lesions [3, 4].

4. What is the role of 18F-FDG PET-CT in T staging of bladder transitional cell carcinoma?
   MRI is considered to be more accurate in T staging of bladder cancer than CT or 18F-FDG PET CT because of its superiority in the assessment of depth of bladder wall infiltration as well as extravesical extension (T3b/4), owing to its high soft tissue contrast resolution. The role of 18F-FDG PET/CT is limited in evaluating primary bladder lesions because tumors are obscured by physiologic intravesical urinary activity [3–5].

© The Author(s), under exclusive license to Springer Nature Switzerland AG 2026
S. Raja et al., *Question and Answers in PET/CT*,
https://doi.org/10.1007/978-3-032-00821-3_14

5. What is the role of 18F-FDG PET-CT in N staging of bladder transitional cell carcinoma?

   Despite its high specificity, routine use of 18F-FDG PET-CT is not recommended in detecting bladder cancer lymph nodal metastases because of its low sensitivity and lack of superiority over MRI [6, 7]. However, it can assess N3 common iliac (N3) lymph nodes when MRI findings are equivocal.

6. What is the role of 18F-FDG PET-CT in M staging of bladder transitional cell carcinoma?

   18F-FDG PET-CT is useful in detecting non-regional nodal and distant metastases of muscle-invasive bladder cancer during staging and restaging [8].

7. What is the role of 18F-FDG PET-CT in the assessment of treatment response in bladder transitional cell carcinoma?

   Initial data show that 18F-FDG PET-CT may be useful in the treatment response evaluation of transitional cell bladder cancer as it can differentiate responders and non-responders to neoadjuvant chemotherapy. However, more studies are needed to validate these observations [9, 10].

8. What are the sensitivity and specificity of 18F-FDG PET-CT in bladder cancer?

   The sensitivity and specificity of 18-FDG PET-CT in detecting urinary bladder cancer are 80% and 84%, respectively [4].

9. What are the sensitivity and specificity of 18F-FDG PET-CT in the assessment of nodal disease in bladder cancer?

   The pooled sensitivity and specificity of 18F-FDG PET-CT in the assessment of nodal disease are 57% and 95%, respectively [6].

10. What are the sensitivity and specificity of 18F-FDG PET-CT in the assessment of distant metastasis in bladder cancer?

    The pooled sensitivity and specificity of 18F-FDG in assessing distant metastases in bladder cancer are 82% and 89%, respectively [8].

11. What are the common pitfalls of 18F-FDG PET-CT in imaging bladder cancer?

    The most common pitfall of 18F-FDG PET-CT in imaging bladder cancer is interference with excreted urinary activity, making interpretation suboptimal.

    Other pitfalls include normal physiologic activity in the bowel, ovaries, endometrium, blood vessels, bladder diverticula, pelvic kidneys, urinary diversions, and so on [11].

12. What are the methods to overcome interference by physiological urinary tracer activity?

    Methods used to overcome interference by physiological urinary tracer activity are late imaging after good hydration and voiding, dual-phase imaging, catheterization, bladder irrigation, forced diuresis, and early dynamic images [5].

13. What are the common false-positive 18F-FDG PET-CT findings in bladder cancer?

    Common false-positive 18F-FDG PET-CT findings in bladder cancer imaging include normal physiologic activity in the urinary tract, bowel, ovaries, endometrium, blood vessels, bladder diverticula, pelvic kidneys, urinary diversions, and so on. In addition, various artifacts such as misregistration artifact, partial volume effect, attenuation correction artifact, and truncation artifact can result in false positives and misregistration artifacts [11, 12].

14. What are the common false-negative 18F-FDG PET-CT findings in bladder cancer?
    (a) Lymph nodes/lesions obscured by physiological tracer activity in the urinary tract, bowel, and reproductive system.
    (b) Small-sized lesions/lymph nodes (smaller than the resolution of the PET scanner).
    (c) Artifacts like misregistration artifacts and so on [5, 12]

15. What are non-FDG tracers in the imaging of bladder cancer?

    To improve PET's sensitivity, various radiotracers that are not excreted in the urine have been tested to evaluate bladder cancer. These are

    (a) 11C choline
    (b) 11C acetate
    (c) 11C methionine
    (d) 18F sodium fluoride is also used to identify skeletal lesions [5].

16. What are the advantages and limitations of 18F-FDG PET-CT in bladder cancer?

    Advantages: 18F-FDG PET-CT is useful in staging and restaging muscle-invasive bladder cancer, particularly in detecting distant metastases. It provides an alternative imaging test for patients with contraindications to MRI and intravenous iodinated contrast administration.

    Limitations: A significant limitation of 18F-FDG PET-CT is interference by urinary tracer activity. This can be overcome by optimizing the imaging protocol by including enforced diuresis, bladder catheterization irrigation, and so on. Its role in treatment response evaluation is yet to be studied [5].

References

1. Kaufman DS, Shipley WU, Feldman AS. Bladder cancer. Lancet. 2009;374:239.
2. Eble JN, Sauter G, Epstein JI, Sesterhenn IA. Pathology and genetics of tumours of the urinary system and male genital organs. Lyon: IARC Press; 2004. p. 143.
3. Bouchelouche K, Choyke PL. PET/computed tomography in renal, bladder, and testicular cancer. PET Clin. 2015;10(3):361–74.
4. Wang N, Jiang P, Lu Y. Is fluorine-18 fluorodeoxyglucose positron emission tomography useful for detecting bladder lesions? A meta-analysis of the literature. Urol Int. 2014;92(2):143–9.
5. Bouchelouche K, Turkbey B, Choyke PL. PET/CT and MRI in bladder cancer. J Cancer Sci Ther. 2012;S14(1):7692.

6. Soubra A, Hayward D, Dahm P, et al. The diagnostic accuracy of 18F-fluorodeoxyglucose positron emission tomography and computed tomography in staging bladder cancer: a single-institution study and a systematic review with meta-analysis. World J Urol. 2016;34(9):1229–37.
7. Salminen AP, Jambor I, Syvanen KT, Bostrom PJ. Update on novel imaging techniques for the detection of lymph node metastases in bladder cancer. Minerva Urol Nefrol. 2016;68(2):138–49.
8. Lu YY, Chen JH, Liang JA, et al. Clinical value of FDG PET or PET/CT in urinary bladder cancer: a systemic review and meta-analysis. Eur J Radiol. 2012;81:2411.
9. Mertens LS, Fioole Bruining A, van Rhijn BW, et al. FDG positron emissionTomography/computerizedtomography for monitoring the response of pelvic lymph node metastasis to neoadjuvant chemotherapy for bladder cancer. J Urol. 2013;189:1687.
10. van de Putte EEF, Vegt E, Mertens LS, et al. FDG-PET/CT for response evaluation of invasive bladder cancer following neoadjuvant chemotherapy. Int Urol Nephrol. 2017; [Epub ahead of print]
11. Subhas N, Patel PV, Pannu HK, Jacene HA, Fishman EK, Wahl RL. Imaging of pelvic malignancies with in-line FDG PET-CT: case examples and common pitfalls of FDG PET. Radiographics. 2005;25(4):1031–43.
12. Corrigan AJ, Schleyer PJ, Cook GJ. Pitfalls and artifacts in the use of PET/CT in oncology imaging. Semin Nucl Med. 2015;45(6):481–99.

Thyroid Cancer

15

1. When is the risk of malignancy associated with incidental focal thyroid uptake on ^{18}F-fluorodeoxyglucose (18F-FDG) positron emission tomography (PET)-computed tomography (CT)?

    The quoted risk of malignancy is 24–36%.

2. What are the common indications of 18F-FDG PET-CT in thyroid cancer?
    (a) Patients with TENIS (thyroglobulin-elevated negative iodine scintigraphy) syndrome with suspected recurrent disease
    (b) Initial staging of poorly differentiated thyroid carcinoma and invasive Hürthle cell carcinoma
    (c) As a prognostic tool in patients with metastatic disease
    (d) Treatment response evaluation of metastatic or locally invasive disease
    (e) Postoperative medullary thyroid cancer (MTC) patients with high serum calcitonin levels with suspected recurrent disease
    (f) Evaluation of anaplastic thyroid carcinoma (ATC) at staging, early treatment response evaluation, and follow-up [1–3]

3. What are the sensitivity and specificity of 18F-FDG thyroid cancer?

    Most well-differentiated thyroid carcinomas are relatively slow-growing and can be FDG-negative. Therefore, the role of FDG PET/CT in the management of patients with differentiated thyroid cancer (DTC) is primarily limited to postoperative follow-up.

    (a) DTC: post thyroidectomy (TENIS) with sensitivity and specificity of 83% and 84%, respectively [4]
    (b) Hürthle cell carcinoma: a multicenter study found 18F-FDG PET CT to have a sensitivity of 92% and a specificity of 95% [5]
    (c) ATC: consistent high FDG uptake is seen, with a quoted sensitivity of 99.6% [6]

4. What are the sensitivity and specificity of 18F-FDG in the assessment of recurrent disease or distant metastasis?
   (a) DTC: 18F-FDG PET/CT has sensitivity and specificity of 79.4% and 79.4%, respectively, in assessing recurrent disease or distant metastasis [7].
   (b) MTC: For recurrent MTC detection, the lowest sensitivity is found in MEN IIA patients, 23% (0% when calcitonin <2000 pg/mL). Per-patient sensitivity increases from 44.1% to 50% when patients with MEN IIA syndrome are excluded [8].

5. What are the common false-positive 18F-FDG PET-CT findings in thyroid cancer?
   (a) Reactive or infective lymph nodes
   (b) Inflammatory/infective soft tissue or skeletal lesions
   (c) Brown fat uptake
   (d) Injection artifact/clot [9]

6. What are the common false-negative 18F-FDG PET-CT findings in thyroid cancer?
   (a) Most well-differentiated thyroid carcinomas are relatively slow-growing and can be FDG-negative
   (b) Small size of the lesion
   (c) Scarce cellularity of the lesion [1, 9, 10]

7. What are the non-FDG PET tracers in imaging thyroid cancer?
   (a) I-124.
   (b) 68Ga-labeled somatostatin analogs (DOTA-Tyr3-octreotate (DOTATATE)/ DOTA-1-Nal3-octreotide (DOTANOC)/DOTA-d-Phe1-Tyr3-octreotide (DOTATOC))
   (c) 18F-DOPA for MTCs [10]

8. What is the role of 18F-FDG PET-CT in the management of thyroid cancer?
   18F-FDG PET-CT is useful in the assessment of poorly DTC, invasive Hürthle cell carcinoma, anaplastic thyroid cancer, and postoperative cases of differentiated (TENIS) and medullary (patients with high calcitonin levels) thyroid cancers.
   In addition, it carries prognostic value, as it has been inferred that

   • FDG uptake is associated with worse prognosis and aggressive tumor in DTC and
   • SUV >18 and FDG uptake volume > 300 mL in Hüthle cell carcinoma are associated with significantly worse 6-month survival rates [10]

9. What is the cost-effectiveness of 18F-FDG PET-CT thyroid cancer?
   18F-FDG PET-CT is not cost-effective in the routine evaluation of DTC patients. As it is a slow-growing tumor, it may not detect all the lesions compared to cheaper I-131 WB scintigraphy and SPECT/CT [11].

10. What are the advantages and limitations of 18F-FDG PET-CT in thyroid cancer?

Advantages: FDG PET/CT is useful in the evaluation of aggressive thyroid cancers such as anaplastic thyroid cancer, invasive Hürthle cell cancer, and poorly differentiated cancer, as well as in dedifferentiating DTC patients (TENIS) and postoperative cases of MTC with high calcitonin levels.

Limitations: Most well-differentiated thyroid carcinomas are relatively slow-growing and can be FDG-negative. Therefore, the role of FDG PET/CT in the initial management of DTC is limited. Since 18F-FDG is a non-specific tracer, infective and inflammatory lesions may produce false positive findings [9, 10].

11. What is the impact of FDG-PET findings on patient management?

It identifies disease in TENIS patients or MTC patients with increased calcitonin levels and guides further treatment.

It identifies additional disease sites in aggressive thyroid cancers, thereby changing management [1–3, 10].

References

1. Haugen BR, Alexander EK, Bible KC, et al. 2015 American Thyroid Association management guidelines for adult patients with thyroid nodules and differentiated thyroid cancer. Thyroid. 2016;26:1–133.
2. Wells SA Jr, Asa SL, Dralle H, et al. Revised American Thyroid Association guidelines for the management of medullary thyroid carcinoma. Thyroid. 2015;25:567–610.
3. Smallridge RC, Ain KB, Asa SL, et al. American Thyroid Association guidelines for management of patients with anaplastic thyroid cancer. Thyroid. 2012;22:1104–39.
4. Dong M-J, Liu Z-F, Zhao K, et al. Value of 18F-FDG-PET/PET-CT in differentiated thyroid carcinoma with radioiodine-negative whole-body scan: a meta-analysis. Nucl Med Commun. 2009;30:639–50.
5. Riemann B, Uhrhan K, Dietlein M, et al. Diagnostic value and therapeutic impact of 18F-FDGPET/CT in differentiated thyroid cancer: results of a German multicentre study. Nuklearmedizin. 2013;52:1–6.
6. Poisson T, Deandreis D, Leboulleux S, et al. 18F-fluorodeoxyglucose positron emission tomography and computed tomography in anaplastic thyroid cancer. Eur J Nucl Med Mol Imaging. 2010;37:2277–85.
7. Haslerud T, Brauckhoff K, Reisæter L. F18-FDG-PET for recurrent differentiated thyroid cancer: a systematic meta-analysis. Acta Radiol. 2016;57:1193–200.
8. Skoura E, Datseris IE, Rondogianni P, et al. Correlation between calcitonin levels and [18F]FDGPET/CT in the detection of recurrence in patients with sporadic and hereditary medullary thyroid cancer. ISRN Endocrinol. 2012;2012:375231.
9. Long NM, Smith CS. Causes and imaging features of false positives and false negatives on F-PET/CT in oncologic imaging. Insights. Imaging. 2011;2:679–98.
10. Marcus C, Whitworth PW, Surasi DS, Pai SI, Subramaniam RM. PET/CT in the Management of Thyroid Cancers. AJR Am J Roentgenol. 2014;202:1316–29.
11. He X, Wang X, Yu J, Ma C. Is it practical and cost effective to detect differentiated thyroid carcinoma metastases by 18F-FDG PET/CT, by 18F-FDG SPET/CT or by 131I SPET/CT? Hell J Nucl Med. 2015;18:2–4.

1. What is the definition, types of Neuroendocrine tumours (NETs) and their salient features?

    1. Neuroendocrine Tumours originate from the neuroendocrine cells, which are found throughout the body and produce hormones [1].
    2. NETs are classified according to their anatomical site of origin, with the vast majority arising in the Gastroenteropancreatic (GEP) or Bronchopulmonary (BP) tracts [1–3].
    3. NETs are subclassified according to the embryological origin of their site as foregut, midgut or hindgut tumours [1–3].
    4. NETs of the GI tract and lung are sometimes referred to as carcinoid tumours, although this older term is no longer used [1–3].
    5. Less common NET sites include the genitourinary tract (such as the kidney, urinary bladder, cervix, ovaries, uterus, prostate and testes), the adrenal medulla(phaeochromocytoma) and the parathyroid and pituitary glands (parathyroid and pituitary adenomas) [1–3].
    6. NETs are well differentiated and should be distinguished from poorly differentiated cancers of neuroendocrine origin, which are classed as neuroendocrine carcinomas (NECs) [1–3].
    7. European Neuroendocrine Tumour Society (ENETS)/WHO grading system for GEP-NETs uses two different proliferative indices: the mitotic count (i.e., the number of mitoses per 10 high-power fields [HPFs]) and the Ki-67 index (i.e., the percentage of cells staining positive for the proliferation marker Ki-67) [2].
    8. Low-grade tumours are grade 1 (G1), intermediate-grade tumours are grade 2 (G2) and high-grade tumours are grade 3 (G3) [1–3].
    9. Well-differentiated NETs are usually G1 or G2, whereas poorly differentiated NECs are always G3 [1–3].

© The Author(s), under exclusive license to Springer Nature
Switzerland AG 2026
S. Raja et al., *Question and Answers in PET/CT*,
https://doi.org/10.1007/978-3-032-00821-3_16

10. Gastroenteropancreatic GEP-NETs with a grade 3 (G3) classification are now separated into two distinct entities: well-differentiated G3 neuroendocrine tumours (NETs G3) and poorly differentiated neuroendocrine carcinomas (NECs) [1–3].

11. In the lung, G1 and G2 tumours are also referred to as 'typical carcinoids' and 'atypical carcinoids', respectively [1–3].

2. What is the Role of Somatostatin receptors in NETs?

Somatostatin receptors (SSTRs) are naturally occurring receptors on cell surfaces that somatostatin, a hormone, binds to. Somatostatin receptor (SSTR) expression is a key feature of well-differentiated neuroendocrine tumours (NETs). There are five subtypes of SSTRs (SSTR1–5), and tumours often express one or more of these subtypes. Radiolabelled somatostatin receptor-based imaging is performed to assess these receptors. Most well-differentiated neuroendocrine tumours (NETs) express high levels of somatostatin receptors, particularly subtypes 2 and 5 [4, 5].

3. How are NETs categorized?

NETs can be categorized based on multiple features, including primary site, stage, differentiation, grade, and SSTR expression. In general, Well-differentiated NETs morphologically resemble endocrine cells of origin. Poorly differentiated neuroendocrine carcinomas are highly aggressive malignancies that tend to express SSTRs weakly [4, 5].

4. What are the sites of metastases from NETs?

In general, Metastatic NETs of different primary sites are quite distinct. Midgut (e.g Ileal or ileocecal) primaries have high propensity to metastasize to mesenteric lymph nodes (often with desmoplastic features), liver, and, less commonly, peritoneum, ovaries, and bone. Metastatic pancreatic NETs also tend to metastasize to the liver and are generally more aggressive than midgut NETs [4, 5].

5. What is the role of Computed tomography (CT) in NETs?

CT scanning of the neck, thorax, abdomen and pelvis is the standard cross-sectional imaging method for the diagnosis, staging and follow-up of patients with NETs. Multiphasic CT allows anatomical assessment of venous and arterial involvement of the tumour to determine surgical resection which is especially relevant in pancreatic NETs and mesenteric masses from intestinal NETs. CT is particularly useful for detection of hepatic metastases (sensitivity, 75–100%; specificity, 83–100%) but is less sensitive for evaluation of nodal disease and bone metastases [6–9].

6. What is the role of Magnetic resonance imaging (MRI) in NETs?

MRI is being increasingly used as an initial imaging investigation in patients with NETs and may be preferred to CT for examination of the liver, pancreas, bone and brain, but is less useful for detection of primary small intestinal NET lesions and nodal metastases. In conventional MRI scans, NETs usually appear as T1- hypointense, T2-hyperintense lesions. Dynamic contrast-enhanced MRI is also recommended, in which NET lesions often appear bright during the arterial phase due to their hypervascularity. For detection of pancreatic NETs, MRI has a reported sensitivity of 54–100% and specificity of 100%; corresponding figures for liver metastases are 70–80% and 98%, respectively. Dynamic and diffusion-weighted MRI is the gold standard for detection of hepatic metastases. MRI is also useful in distinguishing hepatic NET metastases from benign liver lesions such as haemangioma [6–9].

7. What is the role of Endoscopic ultrasonography in NETs?

Endoscopic ultrasonography has high sensitivity (82–93%) and specificity (86–95%) for diagnosis of pancreatic NETs but involves a more invasive investigation than CT or MRI scanning. It also allows histological sampling of pancreatic and duodenal NETs via fine-needle or core biopsy acquisition. The sensitivity of ultrasonography can be improved by use of contrast enhancement [6–9].

8. What positron emission tomography (PET) tracers are used in imaging of neuroendocrine tumors (NETs)?
   a. ^{68}Ga-labeled somatostatin analogs (SSAs)/DOTA (1,4,7,10-tetraazacyclo-dodecane-1,4,7,10-tetraacetic acid) peptides (^{68}Ga-DOTATOC (DOTA-d-Phe1-Tyr3-octreotide), ^{68}Ga-DOTATATE (DOTA-Tyr3-octreotate) and ^{68}Ga-DOTANOC (DOTA-1-Nal3-octreotide))
   b. ^{18}F-fluorodihydroxyphenylalanine (^{18}F-FDOPA)
   c. ^{124}I-metaiodobenzylguanidine
   d. β-[^{11}C]-5-hydroxy-L-tryptophan
   e. ^{68}Ga NOTA-exendin-4
   f. ^{18}F-Flourodeoxy glucose (18F-FDG) [10–12]
   g. ^{18}F-meta-fluorobenzylguanidine [13]

9. What is the role of ^{68}Ga- DOTA peptide PET-computed tomography (CT) in NETs?
   a. Localize primary tumor and detect metastatic disease (staging) sites
   b. Follow up patients with known disease to detect residual, recurrent, or progressive disease (restaging)
   c. Determine somatostatin receptor (SSTR) status visually and using semiquantitative parameters like standardized uptake value
   d. Select patients with metastatic disease for SSTR radionuclide therapy (peptide receptor radionuclide therapy /PRRT [14, 15]

10. What are pheochromocytomas and paragangliomas (PGLs)?

Pheochromocytomas and PGLs are collectively named PPGLs. These NETs arise from pluripotent neural crest stem cells associated with the sympathetic and parasympathetic divisions of the autonomic nervous system. They are benign and slow-growing. However, metastasis and malignant degeneration can occur.

- Sympathetic axis: adrenal medulla, chromaffin cells located in the posterior mediastinum (periaortic regions) or retroperitoneum. May hyper-secrete catecholamines and hence clinical symptoms.
- Parasympathetic ganglia: head and neck, anterior/middle mediastinum. Mostly non-secretary (only 5% are norepinephrine-secreting) and found incidentally or revealed by symptoms of compression or infiltration of the adjacent structures.

   PGL is the term used to describe any sympathetic or parasympathetic extra-adrenal tumors, whereas the WHO classifies pheochromocytomas as adrenal PGL [16].

11. What are the genetic and syndromic association with pheochromocytomas and PGLs?
   a. Solitary pheochromocytomas: 5–10% are hereditary
   b. Multiple pheochromocytomas or a combination of pheochromocytoma with synchronous or metachronous extra-adrenal PGL: in 70% of cases, there is an association with genetic mutations, of which the succinate dehydrogenase subunit B (SDHB) mutation is associated with a higher risk of aggressive behavior due to metastatic disease.

   - Pseudohypoxic cluster: activation of hypoxia-induced factors leading to inhibition of oxidative phosphorylation and activation of glycolytic pathway via the Warburg effect, for example, SDHB, C, D, AF2, Von Hippel-Lindau disease (VHL)
   - Kinase signaling subgroup: MEN2 and NF1

   c. Pheochromocytomas may coexist with other tumor types in MEN2A, MEN2B, VHL, and NF1
   d. Extra-adrenal PGLs may occur in other neuroendocrine syndromes such as Carney-Strakakis syndrome and Carney's triad [16, 17]

12. What is the clinical application of ^{68}Ga-DOTA peptide PET-CT in pheochromocytomas and PGLs?
   PET tracers supersede somatostatin-based imaging with 111In DTPA Pentetreotide (OctreoScanTM) single-photon emission computed tomography/CT [16, 18]. There is limited data on using 68Ga-DOTA peptide PET-CT for primary pheochromocytomas and PGLs. Loss of somatostatin receptor positivity is thought to be associated with a certain level of functional dedifferentiation [19]; however, overall, 68Ga-DOTA peptide PET-CT is reported to be more sensitive than 123/131 meta-iodobenzylguanidine (MIBG) scintigraphy [16, 20].
   Molecular and anatomic imaging (CT/magnetic resonance imaging (MRI)) is often required. Somatostatin cell surface receptor (SSR) type 2 is the most overexpressed subtype. SSR type 1 is also strongly expressed in some PGLs. Other subtypes are slightly or not expressed. The three DOTA peptides all show a high affinity for SSR type 2.

Reporters should remember that the Krenning scale is not validated for 68Ga-DOTA peptide PET-CT. Instead, uptake intensity is graded as mild, moderate, or intense, corresponding to faint, intensity less than, equal to, or greater than the liver.

13. What are the sensitivity and specificity of ^{68}Ga-DOTA (1,4,7,10-tetraazacyclo-dodecane-1,4,7,10-tetraacetic acid) peptide PET-CT in imaging pheochromo-cytomas and PGLs?

There is insufficient data to compare ^{68}Ga-DOTA peptide PET-CT with ^{18}F-FDOPA PET-CT. Pooled detection rate for ^{68}Ga-DOTA peptide PET-CT from a recent systematic review and meta-analysis was 93%, which is significantly higher ($P < 0.001$ for all) than ^{18}F-FDOPA PET-CT, ^{18}F-FDG PET-CT, and $^{123/131}$MIBG scintigraphy [16, 20], with additional lesions identified only on ^{68}Ga-DOTA peptide PET-CT.

14. What are the recommended PET radiotracers for pheochromocytomas and PGLs? [16]

- Sporadic non-metastatic, including rarely occurring non-hypersecreting, pheochromocytomas: 18F-FDOPA PET-CT (and 123MIBG (meta-iodoben-zylguanidine) scintigraphy) is adequate for confirmation. 18F-FDG PET-CT, on the other hand, provides genotype information linked to tumor behavior, such as the SDHB mutation.
- Head and neck PGLs (HNPGL): 18F-FDOPA or 68Ga-DOTA peptide PET-CT. 68Ga-DOTA peptide PET-CT is superior at identifying small lesions overlooked by 18F-FDOPA. In SDHx-related HNPGLs, 18F-FDG PET-CT is complementary to 18F-FDOPA in detecting additional thoracic/abdominal PGLs.
- Retroperitoneal, extra-adrenal, non-metastatic PGLs: once PGL is confirmed, the multiplicity of extra-adrenal localizations can be investigated with 18F-FDOPA and 68Ga-DOTA peptide. 68Ga-DOTA peptide PET-CT is preferred, particularly for SDHx mutations.
- Metastatic PGLs:

- 68Ga-DOTA PET-CT is preferred due to its superiority over 18F-FDOPA regardless of genetic background and the ability to allow PPRT planning.
- 18F-FDOPA PET-CT is a second-line imaging modality when SDHB mutations are absent or when the genetic status is unknown.
- 18F-FDG PET-CT can be considered for SDHB-associated metastatic pheochromocytomas and PGLs.

- If available, PET tracer 124I MIBG can be considered for its theranostic value.
- VHL and RET (MEN2)-associated pheochromocytomas and PGLs: limited data are available for this cohort of patients. Functional imaging is rarely required for MEN2 pheochromocytoma. These tumors are seldom metastatic (<5%). The exceptions are extra-adrenal tumors and pheochromocytomas larger than 5 cm. If an adrenal lesion is not found, 18F-FDOPA PET-CT, 18F-FDG PET-CT, and MRI can be performed preoperatively.

- Screening for SDHx mutations

- SDHD and SDHB mutations cause autosomal dominant diseases; however, disease penetrance varies. Paternally inherited SDHD and SDHB mutation penetrance is >80% and 20–40%, respectively. More frequent and complete follow-up imaging is required; however, no agreed algorithms exist.

15. What are the predictors for metastases and the common metastatic sites of pheochromocytomas and PGLs?

Predictors: PPGL tumor >5 cm, noradrenergic phenotype, dopaminergic phenotype, familial PPGLs (especially SDHB and SDHA), young age at initial diagnosis, multiple tumors, and recurrent disease.

Common metastatic sites: Bone, lymph nodes, liver, and lungs [17].

16. What is ^{68}Ga-DOTA peptide imaging?

SSTRs are found in various tissues, including the gastrointestinal tract and brain. SSTRs are also expressed in numerous tumors, such as NETs (carcinoid, insulinoma, pheochromocytoma, etc.), lung cancer, meningioma, and lymphoma.

SSAs have been developed to target somatostatin receptors (SSRs). These SSAs can be radiolabeled to image somatostatin receptor expression for theranostic purposes. Three well-established SSAs are conjugated to DOTA and labeled with 68Ga (DOTATATE, DOTATOC, and DOTANOC). DOTATATE has a 10-fold higher and selective affinity to the SSR2 receptor. DOTATOC binds to SSR2 and SSR5, whereas DOTATNOC is selective toward SSR2, SSR3, and SSR5.

The imaging carries prognostic and therapeutic information (PRRT), and the theranostic concept allows targeted precision and personalized medicine [18].

17. What are common patient preparations required before ^{68}Ga-DOTA peptide imaging?

No specific patient preparation is warranted before 68Ga-DOTA peptide PET-CT scanning. Empirical evidence calls for imaging on the day(s) preceding the subsequent administration of SSAs, hence discontinuing short- and long-acting SSAs for 1 day or 3 weeks, respectively. Patients are encouraged to void before image acquisition to reduce the background noise and the radiation dose to the kidneys and bladder [16, 21].

18. What is the normal biodistribution in ^{68}Ga-DOTA peptide PET-CT imaging?

68Ga-DOTA-peptides physiologic uptake areas are the pituitary gland, spleen, liver, adrenal glands, thyroid (very mild uptake), and the urinary tract (kidneys and urinary bladder). Intense accumulation is seen in the spleen and accessory splenic tissue. Hepatic uptake is less intense than the spleen. Pancreatic uptake is variable, but most concentrated in the uncinate process. Prostate and glandular breast tissue may show diffuse low-grade uptake. [16, 22]

19. What are common causes of false-negative results in ^{68}Ga-DOTA-peptide imaging?

False-negative causes for ^{68}Ga-DOTA-peptide PET-CT imaging include small lesion size (<5 mm) and low/variable SSR expressing NETs such as medullary thyroid cancer (MTC), neuroblastoma, pheochromocytoma, and insulinoma. Excreted tracer in the urinary bladder may mask intra- or perivesical PGLs [15, 16].

20. What are the common causes of false-positive results in ^{68}Ga-DOTA-peptide imaging?

False-positive causes for ^{68}Ga-DOTA-peptide PET-CT imaging include anatomic structures and lesions with expression of receptors.

Physiological uptake in accessory spleen (can be intrapancreatic) and pancreatic uncinate process may mimic a pancreatic NET [15, 16].

Non-NETs that express somatostatin receptors include the following [18]:

- High expression: meningioma
- Low or varying expression: breast carcinoma, melanoma, lymphoma, prostate carcinoma, non-small cell lung cancer, head and neck cancer, sarcoma, renal cell carcinoma, differentiated thyroid carcinoma, and astrocytoma

21. What are the indications for ^{68}Ga-DOTA-peptides PET-CT in the management of NETs? [19]

- Diagnosis and staging: Localize primary tumors and detect sites of metastasis
- Re-staging: Follow-up of patients with known disease to detect residual, recurrent, or progressive disease
- Prognosis: Determine SSTR status (patients with SSTR-positive tumors are more likely to respond to targeted SSA therapy)
- Management decisions: Select patients with metastatic disease for SSTR radionuclide therapy (with ^{177}Lu or ^{90}Y-DOTA-peptides)
- Monitor response to therapy (surgery, radiotherapy, chemotherapy, or PRRT)

22. What are the advantages of ^{68}Ga-DOTA-peptide PET-CT imaging?

68Ga-DOTA-peptides have the highest accuracy in detecting well-differentiated gastroenteropancreatic (GEP) NETs among all the other available PET tracers. It is also useful in selecting potential patients for PRRT. It also provides prognostic information as high 68 Ga-DOTA peptide avidity indicates well differentiation, thereby a more favorable prognosis.

Its production is relatively easy and cost-effective compared to other tracers like 18F-DOPA or 124I-MIBG.

Compared to somatostatin receptor scintigraphy (SRS), 68Ga-DOTA-peptides have a higher spatial resolution and lower physiologic uptake in the liver and bowel and are less time-consuming (2 vs. 4–24 hours) and cost-effective. Dosimetry can be performed better with 68Ga-DOTA-peptides when compared to SRS [15].

23. What are the sensitivity, specificity, and accuracy of ^{68}Ga-DOTA-peptides PET-CT imaging in NETs?

The overall sensitivity and specificity of 68Ga-DOTA-peptides PET-CT for detecting NET range between 90% and 98% and 92% and 98%, respectively [21, 22]. In addition, sensitivity and specificity are much higher for midgut NETs than lung NETs [23]. The tumor uptake depends on the tumor grading, whereby higher-grade NETs tend to have absent or low SSTR expression [24, 25] but increased FDG avidity.

Neuroendocrine neoplasm (MEN)			
MEN with Ki-67 index < 20%		MEN with Ki-67 index > 20%	
NET G1 (low-grade) NETs	NET G2 (intermediate grade) NETs	NET G3 (high-grade) NETs	Neuroendocrine carcinoma (NEC) with Large cells Small cells
Low grade Ki-67 < 3%	Well differentiated Ki-67 3–20%	Well differentiated Ki-67 21–55%	Poorly differentiated Ki-67 >20%

24. What are the approved indications of ^{18}F-DOPA-PET-CT in NETs in Europe? [19]

- Diagnosis:

  – Diagnosis and location of glomus tumors in patients with *SDHD* variant
  – Localization of pheochromocytoma and PGL
  – Diagnosis and localization of insulinomas in hyperinsulinism in infants and children

- Staging of pheochromocytoma and PGL, and well-differentiated NETs of the digestive tract
- Detection of recurrence and residual disease of

  – Pheochromocytoma and PGL
  – MTC with elevated serum levels of calcitonin
  – Well-differentiated NETs of the digestive tract
  – Other NETs of the digestive tract when SRS is negative

25. What are the common patient preparations required before ^{18}F-DOPA-PET-CT imaging?

Fasting for a minimum of 4 hours without limiting water intake. No drug discontinuation is needed. Premedication of carbidopa, a decarboxylase inhibitor aimed to block the aromatic amino acid decarboxylase enzyme, is controversial [19]. It has been suggested that it would mask insulinoma uptake due to reduced pancreatic physiological uptake [26]. Image acquisition can be early (5–10 minutes) or delayed (20–30 minutes or 45–90 minutes).

26. What is the normal biodistribution in ^{18}F-FDOPA-PET-CT imaging?

Basal ganglia, liver, pancreatic uncinate process, and adrenal glands. There is a variable uptake in excretory organs such as the gallbladder and biliary tract, kidneys, ureters, and urinary bladder. The liver, myocardium, and peripheral muscles can see mild uptake. Faint uptake can be seen in the mammary glands, oral cavity, esophagus, and bowel. Tracer uptake in children's growth plates has been reported [19].

27. What are the advantages and limitations of ^{18}F-FDOPA in imaging NETs?

Advantages:
a. 18F-FDOPA has better sensitivity in detecting NETs with low somatostatin receptor expression.
b. It is considered a tracer of choice in detecting recurrent MTC if conventional imaging fails to detect the disease, mainly when calcitonin and CEA doubling times are longer than 24 months and in MEN II patients.
c. 18F-FDOPA is more sensitive in detecting pheochromocytomas and PGLs. It also plays a complementary role in identifying an islet-cell tumor or carcinoid type of GEP-NET where the location of the primary tumor is unknown (even in 68Ga-DOTA peptide imaging).
d. 18F-FDOPA has high tumor-to-background contrast.
e. Low physiologic uptake in normal adrenal glands.

Limitations:
a. 18F-FDOPA is not widely available.
b. It has relatively less sensitivity in a few tumor subtypes, such as MTC with short calcitonin and CEA doubling times or pheochromocytomas/PGLs with a mutation in SDHB, where 18F–FDG seems to be more sensitive [27].

28. What is the role of ^{18}F-FDG-PET-CT in NET?
a. ^{18}F-FDG PET-CT is very sensitive in assessing disease extent in high-grade poorly differentiated (G3) NETs with aggressive behavior, often as part of PRRT workup.
b. It also has a high prognostic value. Tumors with higher metabolic activity (SUVmax) are associated with significantly poorer overall survival.
c. Part of dual SSTR/FDG PET-CT imaging in the assessment of suitability for PRRT
d. ^{18}F-FDG PET-CT is useful in identifying recurrent MTC, particularly when there is clinical evidence of aggressive disease such as high calcitonin level of > 1,000 pg/mL, a short tumor doubling time, an increased CEA level, or high tumor proliferation index (Ki-67).
e. ^{18}F-FDG PET-CT has higher sensitivity in detecting pheochromocytomas/PGLs with a mutation in SDHB [27, 28].

29. What are the pitfalls of ^{18}F-FDG PET-CT imaging in NETs?

18F-FDG PET-CT is not very sensitive in evaluating well-differentiated NETs because of the slow metabolic rate of these tumors. Since it is a non-specific metabolic tracer, it may be falsely positive in infection/inflammation [15, 26].

30. What is the preferred tracer used in evaluating insulinoma?

SSR 2 expression has been found in up to 80% of insuliomas. Limited research utilizing 68Ga-DOTA-peptides showed variable success and should, therefore, be considered as an adjunct when all imaging studies are negative, especially if a focused or minimally invasive surgical approach is preferred [29].

However, these tumors express a high amount of glucagon-like peptide-1 receptor (GLP-1R) on the cell surface. 68Ga-NOTA-exendin-4 PET/CT targeting GLP-1R has shown the highest sensitivity (up to 97.7%) among available techniques such as SRS, CT, MRI, and endoscopic ultrasonography in detecting insulinomas [12].

31. What is the role of PET/CT in the evaluation of medullary carcinoma of thyroid?

18F-FDOPA PET CT is a highly sensitive investigation detecting recurrent MTC (with sensitivity> 95%).

Patients with features of more aggressive disease, such as short calcitonin and CEA doubling times or initially high biomarker concentrations, may be imaged with 18F-FDG or both tracers.

68Ga-DOTA-peptide PET-CT is complementary in detecting recurrent MTC and exploring the possibility of PRRT [28].

References

1. Raphael MJ, Chan DL, Law C, Singh S. Principles of diagnosis and management of neuroendocrine tumours. CMAJ. 2017;189(10):E398–E404.
2. Rindi G, Klimstra DS, Abedi-Ardekani B, et al. A common classification framework for neuroendocrine neoplasms: an International Agency for Research on Cancer (IARC) and World Health Organization (WHO) expert consensus proposal. Mod Pathol. 2018;31(12):1770–86.
3. Modlin IM, Oberg K, Chung DC, et al. Gastroenteropancreatic neuroendocrine tumours. Lancet Oncol. 2008;9(1):61–72.
4. Strosberg J, Al-Toubah T, et al. Sequencing of somatostatin-receptor–based therapies in neuroendocrine tumor patients. J Nucl Med. 2024;65. https://doi.org/10.2967/jnumed.123.265706.
5. Strosberg JR, Weber JM, Feldman M, et al. Prognostic validity of the American Joint Committee on Cancer staging classification for midgut neuroendocrine tumors. J Clin Oncol. 2013;31:420–25.
6. Sundin A, Arnold R, Baudin E, et al. ENETS Consensus Guidelines for the standards of care in neuroendocrine tumors: Radiological, nuclear medicine & hybrid imaging. Neuroendocrinology. 2017;105(3):212–44.
7. Maxwell JE, Howe JR. Imaging in neuroendocrine tumors: an update for the clinician. Int J Endocr Oncol. 2015;2(2):159–68.

8. Tan EH, Tan CH. Imaging of gastroenteropancreatic neuroendocrine tumors. World J Clin Oncol. 2011;2(1):28–43.

9. Zilli A, Arcidiacono PG, Conte D, Massironi S. Clinical impact of endoscopic ultrasonography on the management of neuroendocrine tumors: lights and shadows. Dig Liver Dis. 2018;50(1):6–14.

10. Maffione AM, Karunanithi S, Kumar R, Rubello D, Alavi A. Nuclear medicine procedures in the diagnosis of NET: a historical perspective. PET Clin. 2014;9:1–9.

11. Koopmans KP, Glaudemans AW. Other PET tracers for neuroendocrine tumors. PET Clin. 2014;9:57–62.

12. Luo Y, Pan Q, Yao S, et al. Glucagon-like peptide-1 receptor PET/CT with 68Ga-NOTA-exendin-4 for detecting localizedinsulinoma: a prospective cohort study. J Nucl Med. 2016;57:715–20.

13. Pandit-Taskar N, Zanzonico P, Staton KD, Carrasquillo JA, Reidy-Lagunes D, Lyashchenko S, et al. Biodistribution and dosimetry of (18)F-meta-fluorobenzylguanidine: a first-in-human PET/CT imaging study of patients with neuroendocrine malignancies. J Nucl Med. 2018;59(1):147–53.

14. Virgolini I, Ambrosini V, Bomanji JB, et al. Procedure guidelines for PET/CT tumour imaging with 68Ga-DOTA-conjugated peptides: 68Ga-DOTA-TOC, 68Ga-DOTA-NOC, 68Ga-DOTA-TATE. Eur J Nucl Med Mol Imaging. 2010;37:2004–10. https://doi.org/10.1007/s00259-010-1512-3.

15. Ambrosini V, Fanti S. 68Ga-DOTA-peptides in the diagnosis of NET. PET Clin. 2014;9:37–42.

16. Taïeb D, Hicks RJ, Hindié E, et al. European Association of Nuclear Medicine Practice Guideline/Society of Nuclear Medicine and Molecular Imaging Procedure Standard 2019 for radionuclide imaging of phaeochromocytoma and paraganglioma. Eur J Nucl Med Mol Imaging. 2019;46(10):2112–37. https://doi.org/10.1007/s00259-019-04398-1.

17. Patel M, Tena I, Jha A, Taieb D, Pacak K. Somatostatin Receptors and Analogs in Pheochromocytoma and Paraganglioma: Old Players in a New Precision Medicine World. Front Endocrinol (Lausanne). 2021;29(12):625312. https://doi.org/10.3389/fendo.2021.625312. PMID: 33854479; PMCID: PMC8039528

18. Duan H, Iagaru A, Aparici CM. Radiotheranostics—precision medicine in nuclear medicine and molecular imaging. Nanotheranostics. 2022;6(1):103–17. https://doi.org/10.7150/ntno.64141. PMID: 34976584; PMCID: PMC8671964

19. Bozkurt MF, Virgolini I, Balogova S, et al. Guideline for PET/CT imaging of neuroendocrine neoplasms with 68Ga-DOTA-conjugated somatostatin receptor targeting peptides and 18F-DOPA. Eur J Nucl Med Mol Imaging. 2017;44:1588–601.

20. Chang CA, Pattison DA, Tothill RW, et al. (68)Ga-DOTATATE and (18)F-FDG PET/CT in paraganglioma and pheochromocytoma: utility, patterns and heterogeneity. Cancer Imaging. 2016;16(1):22. Published 2016 Aug 17. https://doi.org/10.1186/s40644-016-0084-2.

21. Taïeb D, Neumann H, Rubello D, et al. Modern nuclear imaging for paragangliomas: beyond SPECT. J Nuclear Med. 2012;53(2):264–74. https://doi.org/10.2967/jnumed.111.098152.

22. Gabriel M, Decristoforo C, Kendler D, et al. 68Ga- DOTA-Tyr3-octreotide PET in neuroendocrine tumors: comparison with somatostatin receptor scintigraphy and CT. J Nucl Med. 2007;48:508–18.

23. Ambrosini V, Campana D, Tomassetti P, et al. 68Galabelled peptides for diagnosis of gastroenteropancreatic NET. Eur J Nucl Med Mol Imaging. 2012;39:S52–60.

24. Skoura E, Michopoulou S. Mohmaduvesh M, et al. The impact of 68Ga-DOTATATE PET/CT imaging on management of patients with neuroendocrine tumors: experience from a national referral center in the United Kingdom. J Nucl Med. 2016;57:34–40.

25. Kayani I, Bomanji JB, Groves A, et al. Functional imaging of neuroendocrine tumors with combined PET/CT using 68Ga-DOTATATE (DOTA-DPhe1,Tyr3- octreotate) and 18F-FDG. Cancer. 2008;112:2447–2455.

26. Kauhanen S, Seppänen M, Nuutila P. Premedication with carbidopa masks positive finding of insulinoma and beta-cell hyperplasia in [(18)F]-dihydroxy-phenyl-alanine positron emission tomography. J Clin Oncol. 2008;26:5307–8. author reply 5308–9

27. Panagiotidis E, Bomanji J. Role of 18F-fluorodeoxyglucose PET in the study of neuroendocrine tumors. PET Clin. 2014;9:43–55.
28. Minn H, Kemppainen J, Kauhanen S, Forsback S, Seppänen M. 18F-fluorodihydroxyphenylalanine in the diagnosis of neuroendocrine tumors. PET Clin. 2014;9:27–36.
29. Nockel P, Babic B, Millo C, Herscovitch P, Patel D, Nilubol N, Sadowski SM, Cochran C, Gorden P, Kebebew E. Localization of Insulinoma Using 68Ga-DOTATATE PET/CT Scan. J Clin Endocrinol Metab. 2017;102(1):195–9. https://doi.org/10.1210/jc.2016-3445. PMID: 27805844; PMCID: PMC6083884

Gynecological Cancers

17

17.1 Endometrial Cancer

1. What are the common indications of ^{18}F-fluorodeoxyglucose (^{18}F-FDG) positron emission tomography (PET)/computed tomography (CT) in endometrial cancer?

   (a) Detection of nodal and distant metastatic disease in locally advanced disease
   (b) Treatment planning
   (c) Assessment of treatment response
   (d) Evaluation of suspected recurrence and restaging
   (e) Predicting prognosis [1, 2]

2. What is the role of ^{18}F-FDG PET/CT in diagnosing endometrial cancer?

   18F-FDG PET/CT has no established role in detecting and local staging endometrial cancer [1, 2], and this is due to physiological endometrial FDG uptake in pre-menopausal women, superior spatial resolution of ultrasound and magnetic resonance imaging (MRI), limited spatial resolution, and low detectability of small lesions with PET/CT.

3. What is the role of ^{18}F-FDG PET/CT in staging endometrial cancer?

   18F-FDG PET/CT is not of value in T staging of endometrial cancer. However, it can be used for N and M staging locally advanced endometrial cancer [1–3].

With Contributions by Dr. Firuz Ibrahim

© The Author(s), under exclusive license to Springer Nature Switzerland AG 2026
S. Raja et al., *Question and Answers in PET/CT*,
https://doi.org/10.1007/978-3-032-00821-3_17

4. What is the role of ^{18}F-FDG PET/CT in re-staging endometrial cancer?

Guidelines suggest that PET/CT has a higher sensitivity and specificity in assessing suspected relapse of endometrial cancer. In the literature, PET/CT is reported to have better accuracy than CT and MR imaging, high sensitivity (92%–100%) and specificity (88%–95%) in the detection of recurrent disease in both symptomatic and asymptomatic patients with endometrial cancer [5, 6].

In addition, 18F-FDG PET/CT results in modifying both diagnostic and treatment plans in 22.6% of patients in a series by Chung et al. [4].

5. What is the role of ^{18}F-FDG PET/CT in the assessment of treatment response in endometrial cancer?

18F-FDG PET/CT may be used for therapy response assessment of locally advanced endometrial cancer. In a clinical trial where 18F-FDG PET/CT was performed at baseline and after 2 and 6 weeks of temsirolimus therapy, changes in total lesion glycolysis after 2 weeks predicted partial response (PR) after 10 weeks. In contrast, a rise in SUVmax between the second and sixth week predicted progression and was associated with worse progression-free survival. In addition, early response evaluation with 18F-FDG PET/CT is useful in predicting subsequent radiological PR and disease progression [7].

6. What is the role of ^{18}F-FDG PET-CT in T staging?

Due to its limited spatial resolution, 18F-FDG PET/CT is not routinely used for T staging of endometrial carcinoma, as it cannot assess small lesions or degree of endometrial and myometrial invasion, which MRI best evaluates. Initial SUVmax of the primary tumor can help as a predictive biomarker but requires improved standardization and validation of metabolic threshold values. Several researchers have suggested that increasing SUVmax and metabolic tumor volume is associated with a more aggressive histologic grade and worse prognosis [8, 9].

7. What is the role of ^{18}F-FDG PET/CT in N staging?

Even though the specificity of 18F-FDG PET/CT is high (>95–100%), sensitivity is relatively low (53–78%) for detecting pelvic metastatic lymph nodes, significantly smaller (<5 mm) and early metastatic lymph nodes [10, 11]. In a study by Sironi et al., 1081 lymph nodes in 47 patients with early-stage cervical cancer were examined. Overall node-based sensitivity, specificity, Positive Predictive Value (PPV), Negative Predictive Value (NPV), and accuracy of 18F-FDG PET/CT in revealing cancer spread irrespective of the size were 72%, 99.7%, 81%, 99.5%, and 99.3%, respectively [12]. Smaller lymph nodes are a particular challenge. A multicenter prospective study performed histological correlation of 237 negative para-aortic lymph nodes on 18F-FDG PET/CT; 12% were found to be falsely negative, especially for lymph nodes of 5 mm or less [13].

8. What is the role of ^{18}F-FDG PET/CT in M staging?

   18F-FDG PET/CT has high accuracy levels in detecting distant metastases in locally advanced endometrial cancer compared to conventional imaging. It can be used to identify unsuspected distant diseases that would obviate the morbidity of a staging operation [1, 2].

9. What are the common pitfalls of ^{18}F-FDG PET/CT in endometrial cancer?

   Physiological cyclical FDG uptake is seen in normal endometrium during the ovulatory and menstrual phases. FDG uptake may be seen in various benign uterine and endometrial pathologies. Physiological excretion of FDG accumulating in the bladder may mask small pelvic masses, parametrial disease, or parametrial nodes in endometrial cancers. Focal ureteric excretion may be misinterpreted as metabolically active metastatic lymph nodes. Conversely, lymph nodes in the expected course of the ureter may be overlooked and misinterpreted as ureteric tracers. Metallic implants/devices can result in attenuation correction artifacts on PET/CT, masking small-volume peritoneal disease. FDG uptake in the urinary and gastrointestinal tract interferes with lesion detection. Inflammatory and infective pelvic pathology may demonstrate FDG uptake, causing false-positive results [14].

10. What are the common false-positive ^{18}F-FDG PET/CT findings in endometrial cancer?

    Common false-positive 18F-FDG PET/CT findings in endometrial cancer are as follows:

   a. Physiological increased FDG uptake in the endometrium during ovulatory and menstrual flow phases
   b. Endometrial uptake in patients on oral contraceptive pills
   c. Tamoxifen used for breast cancer treatment causes non-tumoral endometrial low-intensity FDG uptake and thickening (polyps, hyperplasia)
   d. Increased FDG uptake has been described in uterine submucosal leiomyomas, endometrial hyperplasia and polyps, and pyometra
   e. FDG tracer uptake in the urinary and gastrointestinal tract also interferes with lesion detection in the abdominal/pelvic region [14]

11. What are the common false-negative ^{18}F-FDG PET/CT findings in endometrial cancer?

    Physiological excretion of FDG accumulating in the bladder may mask small pelvic masses, parametrial disease, or parametrial nodes in endometrial cancers [14]. Small (≤5 mm) lymph nodes [13].

12. What are the non-FDG tracers in imaging endometrial cancer
    (a) ^{11}C-methionine
    (b) [11]C -choline
    (c) ^{18}F-fluoro-17-beta-estradiol (FES) [15]

13. What is the role of ^{18}F-FDG PET/CT in radiotherapy planning in endometrial cancer?

Only limited data is available on the role of ^{18}F-FDG PET/CT in post-surgical radiotherapy planning of endometrial cancer.

14. What are the advantages and limitations of ^{18}F-FDG PET/CT in endometrial cancer?

Advantages: Initiation of treatment can be facilitated by early detection of recurrent disease by PET/CT in asymptomatic patients and may improve patient quality of life.

Although the sensitivity of 18F-FDG PET/CT in detecting lymph nodal metastases is insufficient to forego surgical lymphadenectomy in most patients, the high specificity may allow a tailored approach in poor surgical candidates [16–18].

The detection of distant diseases that may not be apparent in standard staging.

Limitations: Poor spatial resolution and respiratory motion artifact limit identifying sub-diaphragmatic peritoneal disease, sub-centimeter peritoneal deposits, and lung nodules. Various pitfalls such as inflammatory and infective pelvic pathologies and physiological uptake in the genitourinary and gastrointestinal tract can cause false positive/false negative results [19].

17.2   Ovarian Cancer

1. What are the common indications of ^{18}F-FDG PET/CT in ovarian cancer?
   (a) Detection of nodal and distant metastases.
   (b) Detection of recurrence in patients with CA 125 relapse.
   (c) Response assessment to chemotherapy [1, 2]

2. What is the role of ^{18}F-FDG PET/CT in diagnosing ovarian cancer?

18F-FDG PET/CT has no role in the diagnosis of ovarian cancer. Although primary ovarian neoplasm will display FDG uptake, the overlap of patterns of metabolic uptake with benign lesions, variable sensitivity and specificity, and the cost of the scan dictate that the procedure provides no additional value. The likelihood of malignant disease increases with increasing SUV Max. With a cut-off of 2.5 SUVmax, the sensitivity and specificity for detecting a malignant ovarian lesion are 80.6% to 82.4% and 76.9% to 94.6%, respectively [1, 2, 20, 21].

3. What is the role of ^{18}F-FDG PET/CT in staging ovarian cancer?

^{18}F-FDG PET/CT is not routinely recommended for initial staging. CT of the chest, abdomen, and pelvis and pelvic MRI have been the imaging techniques of choice in the primary staging of ovarian cancer. A few studies have shown that FDG PET/CT increases the pre-treatment staging accuracy to

69–75% compared with 53–55% with CT alone. PET/CT is useful in differentiating stage IIIC–IV from other stages with a sensitivity of 100% and specificity of 91%, whereas CT has a sensitivity of 97% and specificity of 64% [22–24].

4. What is the role of ^{18}F-FDG PET/CT in recurrence assessment of ovarian cancer?

The most significant value of 18F FDG PET/CT lies in the high accuracy in detecting residual disease after primary therapy and in identifying recurrent disease, with a pooled sensitivity and specificity of 89% and 90%, respectively. The high accuracy in detecting recurrent disease makes PET/CT a valuable tool for selecting patients who may benefit from secondary cytoreductive surgery. Fulham et al. found that evidence of recurrent ovarian cancer on FDG PET/CT can precede CT findings by 6 months [1, 2, 25].

5. What is the role of ^{18}F-FDG PET/CT in the assessment of treatment response in ovarian cancer?

18F-FDG PET/CT is useful in predicting early response to neoadjuvant chemotherapy in advanced ovarian cancer. It provides prognostic information, as the overall survival is better in metabolic responders than in non-responders [1, 2, 26].

6. What is the role of ^{18}F-FDG PET/CT in T staging?

^{18}F-FDG PET CT has no role in T staging of ovarian malignancy [1, 2].

7. What is the role of ^{18}F-FDG PET/CT in N staging?

The reported sensitivity, specificity, accuracy, positive predictive value, and negative predictive value of ^{18}F-FDG PET/CT in the detection of nodal metastases is 83.3%, 98.2%, 95.6%, 90.9%, and 96.5%, respectively. The high negative predictive value may allow avoidance of lymphadenectomy, which is associated with increased morbidity and cost [1, 2].

8. What is the role of ^{18}F-FDG PET/CT in M staging?

18-F FDG PET/CT provides an accurate assessment of the extent of the disease, particularly in the mediastinum and supraclavicular region. Many studies have shown that 18F-FDG PET/CT upstages disease, largely due to the identification of supradiaphragmatic metastases not imaged or identified on contrast-enhanced CT [1, 2].

9. What are the common pitfalls of ^{18}F-FDG PET/CT in ovarian cancer?

In the preovulatory phase and luteal cysts, physiological ovarian uptake may be seen in premenopausal patients. FDG tracer uptake in the urinary and gastrointestinal tract interferes with lesion detection in the abdominal/pelvic region. Mucinous ovarian tumors and necrotic lymph nodes may have no or very low FDG uptake and may be missed. Poor spatial resolution and respiratory motion artifact limit the identification of sub-diaphragmatic disease, small-volume peritoneal disease, and small lung lesions [14].

10. What are the common false-positive ^{18}F-FDG PET/CT findings in ovarian cancer?

    In the preovulatory phase and luteal cysts, physiological ovarian uptake may be seen in premenopausal patients. FDG tracer uptake in the urinary and gastrointestinal tract also interferes with lesion detection in the abdominal/pelvic region. A few benign adnexal lesions may show abnormal FDG uptake, including cystadenoma, endometrioma, hydrosalpinx, benign germ cell tumors, cholesterol granuloma, abscess, and thecomas. Hyperstimulated ovaries due to gonadotropin stimulation also show increased FDG uptake [14, 27].

11. What are the common false-negative ^{18}F-FDG PET/CT findings in ovarian cancer?

    FDG-PET/CT can be falsely negative in small, necrotic, mucinous, cystic, or low-grade tumors. Another limitation is the ability of FDG-PET/CT to identify lesions less than 1 cm, particularly those smaller than 5 mm [14, 27].

12. What are the non-FDG tracers in imaging ovarian cancer?
    (a) ^{11}C- methionine
    (b) ^{11}C-choline [15]

13. What is the role of ^{18}F-FDG PET/CT in radiotherapy planning in ovarian cancer?
    Only limited data is available on the role of 18F-FDG PET/CT in radiotherapy planning of ovarian cancer. Radiotherapy is not a routine ovarian cancer treatment of choice.

14. What are the advantages and limitations of ^{18}F-FDG PET/CT in ovarian cancer?
    Advantages: Useful in detecting distant metastases and peritoneal deposits and in evaluating suspected relapse. It may play a role in the treatment response evaluation of advanced ovarian cancer.

    Limitations: False-negative findings may be seen in mucinous, necrotic, cystic, or low-grade tumors. Due to limited spatial resolution, small lesions might be missed. High cost and limited availability [1, 2].

17.3   Cervical Cancer

1. What are the common indications of ^{18}F-FDG PET/CT in cervical cancer?
   (a) Detection of lymph nodal and distant metastases in locally advanced disease
   (b) Treatment response assessment
   (c) Radiotherapy planning
   (d) Tumor recurrence assessment and Restaging
   (e) Prognosis assessment [1, 2, 28]

2. What is the role of ^{18}F-FDG PET/CT in diagnosing cervical cancer?

   The diagnosis of cervical cancer is based on clinical examination and cervical biopsy. 18F-FDG PET/CT is not useful in diagnosing cervical cancer. 18F-FDG PET/CT has limited spatial resolution to detect small early cancer lesions (Stage IA or IB) [1, 2].

3. What is the role of ^{18}F-FDG PET/CT in staging cervical cancer?

   Due to its limited spatial resolution and low detectability of small lesions and early cancer, 18F-FDG PET/CT has a limited role in T staging. Still, it is useful in assessing lymph nodal and distant metastatic disease [1, 2, 29].

4. What is the role of ^{18}F-FDG PET/CT in re-staging cervical cancer?

   18F-FDG PET/CT is useful in detecting local recurrence and distant metastases (especially in asymptomatic patients) with high diagnostic performance. PET/CT has a high accuracy of 92% in the detection of recurrent disease, with a sensitivity of 82% and specificity of 97% [30].

5. What is the role of ^{18}F-FDG PET/CT in the assessment of treatment?

   18F-FDG PET/CT can be used to monitor treatment response to chemoradiation in advanced cervical cancer patients and provides prognostic information, as the early metabolic response predicts disease-free survival and overall survival [28, 31].

6. What is the role of ^{18}F-FDG PET/CT in T staging?

   Due to the limited spatial resolution, 18F-FDG-PET/CT has poor efficacy for detecting small lesions, including early cancer and assessment of local cancer spread. MRI is preferred when defining local tumor invasion [32].

7. What is the role of ^{18}F-FDG PET/CT in N staging?

   Accurate anatomical localization of involved lymph nodes is essential for FIGO staging and surgical planning. 18F-FDG PET/CT has low detectability of nodal metastases in early cervical cancers, where the pre-test probability is low. However, it is useful in advanced (stage IIB and more) cervical cancer patients in the detection of nodal metastases with a sensitivity of more than 80% (only around 50% for CT and MRI) and specificity of 95% (>90% for CT and MRI) [33, 34, 35]. Nodal detectability is limited by nodal size (~5 mm). Micrometastases cannot be detected.

8. What is the role of ^{18}F-FDG PET/CT in M staging?

   18F-FDG PET/CT is useful for evaluating distant metastases such as distant lymph nodes, bone, and intramuscular metastases. Wong et al. reported a sensitivity of 100%, a specificity of 90%, and an accuracy of 94% of PET to evaluate distant metastases, especially those in unusual sites such as supraclavicular and mediastinal lymph nodes [34]. False-negative metastatic nodal disease has been reported, however.

9. What are the common pitfalls of ^{18}F-FDG PET/CT in cervical cancer?

    Reports of para-aortic lymph node involvement are false negative on 18F-FDG PET/CT. This can be a source of negative outcomes if pelvic chemoradiation or limited pelvic surgery is the treatment choice. Therefore, systematic lymph node dissection for metastatic diagnosis cannot be replaced by FDG PET/CT. Inflammatory and infective pelvic pathology may demonstrate 18F-FDG uptake, thereby causing false-positive results. Focal ureteric excretion may be misinterpreted as metabolically active metastatic lymph nodes. Physiological excretion of FDG accumulating in the bladder may mask small pelvic masses, parametrial disease, or parametrial nodes. Due to limited spatial resolution, small lesions or lymph nodes might be missed. Necrotic lymph nodes might show no FDG uptake [14, 27].

10. What are the common false-positive ^{18}F-FDG PET/CT findings in cervical cancer?

    Inflammatory and infective pelvic pathology may demonstrate 18F-FDG PET/CT uptake, thereby causing false positive results. Focal ureteric excretion may be misinterpreted as metabolically active metastatic lymph nodes [14, 27]. Endometriosis, often found in the retrocervical deep pelvis, can be FDG-avid.

11. What are the common false-negative ^{18}F-FDG PET/CT findings in cervical cancer?

    Physiological excretion of FDG accumulating in the bladder may mask small pelvic masses, parametrial disease, or parametrial nodes in cervical cancer [14, 27].

12. What are the non-FDG tracers in imaging cervical cancer?
    (a) ^{11}C-methionine
    (b) ^{11}C-choline
    (c) [64] Cu-ATSM and 60 Cu-ATSM [15]

13. What is the role of ^{18}F-FDG PET/CT in radiotherapy planning in cervical cancer?

    18F-FDG PET/CT provides information to modify radiation treatment volumes and radiation dose to metabolically positive lymph nodes and allows for image-guided brachytherapy. 18F-FDG-based brachytherapy treatment planning can potentially improve isodose tumor coverage while sparing the critical organs [1].

14. What are the advantages and limitations of ^{18}F-FDG PET/CT in cervical cancer?

    Advantages: 18F-FDG PET/CT is useful in detecting lymph nodal and distant metastases in locally advanced cervical cancer and assessing suspected recurrence. It may play an important role in therapy response assessment and radiotherapy planning.

    Limitations: Due to limited spatial resolution, small lesions might be missed. Necrotic lymph nodes might be FDG-negative. High cost and limited availability [1, 2].

References

1. Hildebrandt MG, Kodahl AR, Teilmann-Jørgensen D, Mogensen O, Jensen PT. [^{18}F]fluorode-oxyglucose PET/computed tomography in breast cancer and gynecologic cancers: a literature review. PET Clin. 2015;10(1):89–104.
2. Brunetti JC, Fludeoxyglucose F. 18 PET-computed tomography: management changes effecting patient outcomes in gynecologic malignancies. PET Clin. 2015;10(3):395–409.
3. Rockall AG, Cross S. The role of FDG PET/CT in gynaecological malignancies. Cancer Imaging. 2012;12:49–65.
4. Chung HH, Kang WJ, Kim JW, Park NH, Song YS, Chung JK, et al. The clinical impact of [(18)F]FDG PET/CT for the management of recurrent endometrial cancer: correlation with clinical and histological findings. Eur J Nucl Med Mol Imaging. 2008;35:1081–8.
5. Ryu SY, Kim K, Kim K, et al. Detection of recurrence by 18F-FDG PET in patients with endometrial cancer showing no evidence of disease. J Korean Med Sci. 2010;25(7):1029–33.
6. Ozcan KP, Kara T, Kaya B, et al. The value of FDG- PET/CT in the post-treatment evaluation of endome- trial carcinoma: a comparison of PET/CT findings with conventional imaging and CA 125 as a tumour marker. Rev Esp Med Nucl Imagen Mol. 2012;31(5):257–60.
7. Boers-Sonderen MJ, de Geus-Oei LF, Desar IM, van der Graaf WT, Oyen WJ, Ottevanger PB, et al. Temsirolimus and pegylated liposomal doxorubicin (PLD) combination therapy in breast, endometrial, and ovarian cancer: phase Ib results and prediction of clinical outcome with FDG-PET/CT. Target Oncol. 2014;9(4):339–47.
8. Nakamura K, Hongo A, Kodama J, Hiramatsu Y. The measurement of SUVmax of the primary tumor is predictive of prognosis for patients with endometrial cancer. Gynecol Oncol. 2011;123:82–7.
9. Nakamura K, Joja I, Fukushima C, Haruma T, Hayashi C, Kusumoto T, et al. The preoperative SUVmax is superior to ADCmin of the primary tumour as a predictor of disease recurrence and survival in patients with endometrial cancer. Eur J Nucl Med Mol Imaging. 2013;40:52–60.
10. Chang MC, Chen JH, Liang JA, et al. 18-F FDG PET or PET/CT for detection of metastatic lymph nodes in patients with endometrial cancer: a systematic review and meta-analysis. Eur J Radiol. 2012;81(11):3511–7.
11. Kitajama K, Murakami K, Yamasaki E, et al. Accuracy of 18F-FDG PET/CT in detecting pelvic and para-aortic lymph node metastases in patients with endometrial cancer. AJR Am J Roentgenol. 2008;190(6):1652–8.
12. Sironi S, Buda A, Picchio M, Perego P, Moreni R, Pellegrino A, et al. Lymph node metastasis in patients with clinical early-stage cervical cancer: detection with integrated FDG PET/CT. Radiology. 2006;238:272–9.
13. Gouy S, Morice P, Narducci F, Uzan C, Martinez A, Rey A, et al. Prospective multicenter study evaluating the survival of patients with locally advanced cervical cancer undergoing laparoscopic para-aortic lymphadenectomy before chemoradiotherapy in the era of positron emission tomography imaging. J Clin Oncol. 2013;31:3026–33.
14. Even-Sapir E. Imaging the normal and abnormal anatomy of the female pelvis using (18) F FDG-PET/CT, including pitfalls and artifacts. PET Clin. 2010;5(4):425–34.
15. Basu S, Kwee TC, Alavi A. PET and PET/CT assessment of gynecologic malignancies: beyond FDG. PET Clin. 2010;5(4):477–82.
16. Signorelli M, Guerra L, Buda A, et al. Role of the integrated FDG PET/CT in the surgical management of patients with high risk clinical early stage endometrial cancer: detection of pelvic nodal metastases. Gynecol Oncol. 2009;115(2):231–5.
17. Park JY, Kim EN, Kim DY, et al. Comparison of the validity of magnetic resonance imaging and positron emission tomography/computed tomography in preoperative evaluation of patients with uterine corpus cancer. Gynecol Oncol. 2008;58(1):24–38.
18. Crivellaro C, Signorelli M, Guerra L, et al. Tailoring systemic lymphadenectomy in high risk clinical early stage endometrial cancer: role of 18F-FDG PET/CT. Gynecol Oncol. 2013;130(2):306–11.

19. Narayanan P, Sahdev A. The role of 18F-FDG PET CT in common gynaecological malignancies. Br J Radiol. 2017;90:20170283.
20. Pandit-Taskar N. Oncologic imaging in gynecologic malignancies. J Nucl Med. 2005;46:1842–50.
21. Kumar R, Alavi A. PET imaging in gynecologic malignancies. Radiol Clin North Am. 2004;42:1155–67.
22. Castellucci P, Perrone AM, Picchio M. Diagnostic accuracy of 18F-FDG PET/CT in characterizing ovarian lesions and staging ovarian cancer: correlation with transvaginal ultrasonography, computed tomography, and histology. Nucl Med Commun. 2007;28:589–95.
23. Kitajama K, Suzki K, Senda M, et al. FDG-PET/CT for diagnosis of primary ovarian cancer. Nucl Med Commun. 2011;32(7):549–53.
24. Tanzaki Y, Kobayashi A, Shiro M, et al. Diagnostic value of preoperative SUVmax on FDG-PET/CT for the detection of ovarian cancer. Int J Gynecol Cancer. 2014;24(3):454–60.
25. Fulham MJ, Carter J, Baldey A, et al. The impact of PET-CT in suspected recurrent ovarian cancer: a prospective multi-Centre study as part of the Australian PET data collection project. Gynecol Oncol. 2009;112:462–8.
26. Avril N, Sassen S, Schmalfeldt B, et al. Prediction of response to Neoadjuvant chemotherapy by sequential F-18-fluorodeoxyglucose positron emission tomography in patients with advanced-stage ovarian cancer. J Clin Oncol. 2005;23:7445–53.
27. Subhas N, Patel PV, Pannu HK, et al. Imaging of pelvic malignancies with in-line FDG PET-CT: case examples and common pitfalls of FDG PET. Radiographics. 2005;25(4):1031–43.
28. Kheiwvan B, Torigian DA, Emamzadehfard S, et al. Update of the role of PET/CT and PET/MRI in the management of patients with cervical cancer. Hell J Nucl Med. 2016;19(3):254–68.
29. Lee, et al. Evaluation of gynecologic cancer with MR imaging, 18F-FDG PET/CT, and PET/MR imaging. J Nuclear Med. 2015;56:436–43.
30. Sharma DN, Rath GK, Kumar R, Malhotra A, Kumar S, Pandjatcharam J, et al. Positron emission tomography scan for predicting clinical outcome of patients with recurrent cervical carcinoma following radiation therapy. J Cancer Res Ther. 2012;8:23–7.
31. Kidd EA, et al. Changes in cervical cancer FDG uptake during chemoradiation and association with response. Int J Radiat Oncol Biol Phys. 2013;85(1):116–22.
32. Sun H, Xin J, Zhang S, et al. Anatomical and functional volume concordance between FDG PET, and T2 and diffusion-weighted MRI for cervical cancer: a hybrid PET/MR study. Eur J Nucl Med Mol Imaging. 2014;41:898–905.
33. Yildirim Y, Sehirali S, Avci ME, etal: Integrated PET/CTfortheevaluation of para-aortic nodal metastasis in locally advanced cervical cancer patients with negative conventional CT findings. Gynecol Oncol 2008; 108: 154–159.
34. Choi HJ, Roh JW, Seo SS, etal: Comparison of the accuracy of magnetic resonance imaging and positron emission tomography/computed tomography in the presurgical detection of lymph node metastases in patients with uterine cervical carcinoma: a prospective study. Cancer 2006; 106: 914–922.
35. Wong T Z etal. Positron emission tomography with 2-deoxy-2-18F fluoro-D-glucose for evaluating local and distant disease in patients with cervical cancer. Mol Imaging Biol 2004; 6(1):55–62.

Head and Neck Cancer

18

1. What are the common indications of ^{18}F-fluorodeoxyglucose (18F-FDG) positron emission tomography (PET)/computed tomography (CT) in head and neck cancer (HNC)?

    The common indications of 18F-FDG PET/CT in HNC are as follows:

    (a) Identification of primary site in histologically confirmed carcinoma of unknown head and neck primary (commonly presenting as neck mass)
    (b) Initial staging of advanced-stage oral cavity, oropharyngeal, hypopharyngeal, glottic, and supraglottic cancers (American Joint Committee on Cancer (AJCC) stage III–IV disease), as well as mucosal melanoma and nasopharyngeal carcinoma
    (c) Assessment of treatment response
    (d) Detection of residual/recurrent tumor
    (e) Radiotherapy planning [1]

2. What is the role of 18F-FDG PET/CT in diagnosing HNC?

    18F-FDG PET/CT is superior to conventional imaging in the localization of the primary site and guiding biopsy site (s) in patients with carcinoma of unknown head and neck primary site. A meta-analysis showed a pooled sensitivity and specificity of 89.3% and 89.5%, compared with 71.6% and 78% for conventional imaging. However, it is considered an adjunct tool but not a substitute for the conventional protocol of pan-endoscopy followed by biopsy. 18F-FDG PET/CT is also helpful in identifying synchronous malignancy, a relatively common occurrence in HNC [2].

With Contributions by Dr. Arun Kumar Reddy Gorla

S. Raja et al., *Question and Answers in PET/CT*, https://doi.org/10.1007/978-3-032-00821-3_18

3. What is the role of 18F-FDG PET/CT in staging HNC?

    18F-FDG PET/CT is recommended in the staging evaluation of advanced stage HNC (stage III–IV oral cavity, oropharyngeal, hypopharyngeal, glottic, and supraglottic cancers, and mucosal melanoma and nasopharyngeal carcinoma) as it has higher sensitivity and specificity in the detection of nodal and distant metastases, thus accurately staging the disease. It is reported that 18F-FDG PET/CT can change clinical management in up to 13.7% of cases [3, 4].

4. What is the role of 18F-FDG PET in re-staging HNC?

    18F-FDG PET/CT can accurately determine residual disease with a very high NPV. Thus, a negative PET/CT study rules out residual viable disease. However, false-positive uptake due to treatment-related inflammation and benign pathologies results in poor PPV. As such, a positive study shall warrant further confirmation by histological evaluation. 18F-FDG PET/CT facilitates patient selection for surgery following chemoradiation [3, 5, 6].

5. What is the role of 18F-FDG PET in the assessment of treatment response in HNC?

    The treatment of advanced-stage HNC often involves multi-modality treatment, including surgery, chemotherapy, and radiotherapy. Due to altered anatomical planes and soft tissue architecture due to treatment-related fibrosis, conventional imaging performs poorly in accurate response evaluation of HNC. 18F-FDG PET/CT performed 3–6 months post-chemo-radiotherapy provides metabolic information, which infers better accuracy in response assessment [7–9].

6. What are the sensitivity and specificity of 18F-FDG PET/CT in the assessment of distant metastasis?

    Pooled sensitivity and specificity in the region of ~88% and ~ 95%, respectively, were reported by Xu et al. in both their meta-analyses of PET/CT for the detection of distant metastases in HNC [10, 11].

7. What is the role of 18F-FDG PET-CT in T staging?

    18F-FDG PET/CT is more sensitive in detecting the primary site than CT alone, especially in superficial tumors (such as tongue, lips, and gingiva) and tumors in locations with indistinct borders and poor enhancement. However, MR imaging scores ahead in specific local soft tissue invasion cases and perineural spread. Hence, 18F-FDG PET/CT is complementary to conventional T staging imaging [3, 9, 12].

8. What is the role of 18F-FDG PET-CT in N staging?

    18F-FDG PET/CT is superior in diagnostic performance compared to conventional imaging for nodal staging of HNC. 18F-FDG PET/CT is demonstrated to have similar specificity but higher per-neck level sensitivity for nodal detection compared to conventional imaging. The increased sensitivity is ascribed to the detection of uptake of involved nodes, which are otherwise considered normal by anatomical criteria [13]. Early studies demonstrated that clinically node-negative (cN0) patients are poor candidates for evaluation by 18F-FDG PET/CT due to the inherent poor resolution, which may not hold with advancements in modern instrumentation [14].

9. What is the role of 18F-FDG PET-CT in M staging?

18F-FDG PET/CT has better diagnostic accuracy in detecting metastatic spread in HNC than conventional imaging. The detection of metastasis can avoid radical curative-intent surgery and the significant morbidity associated. Early and accurate metastatic workups can change the management of up to 13% of patients [2, 10, 11].

10. What are the common pitfalls of 18F-FDG PET-CT in HNC?

Physiological uptake and artifacts are potential pitfalls in 18-FDG PET/CT imaging of HNC, including:

- Lymphoid tissue (Waldeyer's ring), mucosa of the hard and soft palate
- Muscle uptake (extraocular muscles, tongue, muscles of mastication)
- Major and minor salivary gland tracer uptake
- Vocal cord uptake (due to vocalization during the uptake phase)
- Brown adipose tissue tracer uptake
- Artifacts due to dental hardware/implants/motion [15, 16]
- Intense FDG uptake in post-surgical flaps

11. What are the common false-positive 18F-FDG PET-CT findings in HNC?

1. Infective lesions (sinusitis, tonsillitis, pharyngitis) and resultant lymphadenopathy
2. Post-RT/post-surgical sterile inflammation
3. Muscle uptake (secondary to strain)
4. Benign lesions (e.g., granulomas and thyroid adenoma) [16–18]

12. What are the common false-negative 18F-FDG PET-CT findings in HNC?

1. Small lesion/nodal size
2. Poorly FDG-avid histology (poorly glycolytic metabolic phenotype)
3. Proximity to highly FDG-avid organ/lesion (e.g., brain)
4. Artifacts due to patient motion during scan acquisition [17, 18]

13. What is the role of non-FDG tracers in imaging HNC?

Several non-FDG tracers are utilized for biological and molecular profiling of the HNC, including:

- 18F-MISO (misonidazole)/FAZA/60Cu-ATSM/18F-Flortanidazole (HX4) have been investigated in tumor hypoxia evaluation. This tracer has a potential role in identifying radioresistant hypoxic tumors in RT planning (dose painting) and prognostication of treatment response.

- 18F-FET (fluoroethyl tyrosine) has been utilized to assess amino acid metabolism. This tracer has been shown to have better specificity but poor sensitivity compared to 18-F FDG, a potential tracer for response evaluation.
- 18F-FLT (fluorothymidine) is a proliferation marker and can serve as an indication of tumor proliferation. Currently, there are no promising results.
- Immuno-PET (Zr-89 mAb U36)/TKI PET imaging has been described in molecular profiling and targeting of tumors. However, further evaluation and validation are needed [19, 20].

14. What is the role of 18F-FDG PET-CT in radiotherapy planning in HNC?
^{18}F-FDG PET/CT has a role in:

   (a) Improving diagnostic certainty (as compared to CT alone)
   (b) Better delineating tumors in locations with indistinct borders and poor enhancement
   (c) Selecting patients for radical treatment by detecting additional nodal disease [21–23]. PET-based tumor segmentation and target volume determination are proving increasingly promising with the advent of gradient and iterative methods that reduce variability between radiation oncologists [23, 24].

15. What is the cost-effectiveness (CE) of 18F-FDG PET-CT HNC?

Encouraging results are noted in CE analyses of 18F-FDG PET-CT in managing HNC. A systematic review of four studies suggests that it is cost-effective for the indications of staging and restaging of HNC [25]. A recent study based on the PET-NECK trial (a multicenter randomized phase III trial) concluded that including PET/CT in managing advanced HNC after primary CRT reduced lifetime costs and improved outcomes [26].

16. What are the advantages and limitations of FDG PET-CT in HNC?

Advantages: 18F-FDG PET/CT is superior to conventional imaging for identifying unknown head and neck primary sites, staging evaluation of advanced-stage HNC, restaging following treatment, response evaluation following treatment, RT planning, and prognostic stratification [1, 3, 4].

Limitations: Relatively lower sensitivity in evaluating glandular tumors (salivary, thyroid), false-positive uptake in physiological sites, and benign/inflammatory lesions [3, 13, 15].

References

1. Lauridsen JK, Rohde M, Thomassen A. (1)(8)F-fluorodeoxyglucose-positron emission tomography/computed tomography in malignancies of the thyroid and in head and neck squamous cell carcinoma: a review of the literature. PET clinics. 2015;10(1):75–88.
2. Rohde M, Dyrvig AK, Johansen J, et al. 18Ffluoro-deoxy-glucose-positron emission tomography/ computed tomography in diagnosis of head and neck squamous cell carcinoma: a systematic review and meta-analysis. Eur J Cancer. 2014;50(13):2271–9.

3. Tantiwongkosi B, Yu F, Kanard A, Miller FR. Role of (18)F-FDG PET/CT in pre and post treatment evaluation in head and neck carcinoma. World J Radiol. 2014;6(5):177–91.
4. Sheikhbahaei S, Marcus C, Subramaniam RM. 18F FDG PET/CT and head and neck cancer: patient management and outcomes. PET clinics. 2015;10(2):125–45.
5. Andrade RS, Heron DE, Degirmenci B, Filho PA, Branstetter BF, Seethala RR, et al. Posttreatment assessment of response using FDG-PET/CT for patients treated with definitive radiation therapy for head and neck cancers. Int J Radiat Oncol Biol Phys. 2006;65(5):1315–22.
6. Evangelista L, Cervino AR, Chondrogiannis S, Marzola MC, Maffione AM, Colletti PM, et al. Comparison between anatomical cross-sectional imaging and 18F-FDG PET/CT in the staging, restaging, treatment response, and long-term surveillance of squamous cell head and neck cancer: a systematic literature overview. Nucl Med Commun. 2014;35(2):123–34.
7. Kawabe J, Higashiyama S, Yoshida A, Kotani K, Shiomi S. The role of FDG PET-CT in the therapeutic evaluation for HNSCC patients. Jpn J Radiol. 2012;30(6):463–70.
8. Gupta T, Master Z, Kannan S, Agarwal JP, Ghsoh-Laskar S, Rangarajan V, et al. Diagnostic performance of post-treatment FDG PET or FDG PET/CT imaging in head and neck cancer: a systematic review and meta-analysis. Eur J Nucl Med Mol Imaging. 2011;38(11):2083–95.
9. Seitz O, Chambron-Pinho N, Middendorp M, Sader R, Mack M, Vogl TJ, et al. 18F-Fluorodeoxyglucose-PET/CT to evaluate tumor, nodal disease, and gross tumor volume of oropharyngeal and oral cavity cancer: comparison with MR imaging and validation with surgical specimen. Neuroradiology. 2009;51(10):677–86.
10. Xu GZ, Zhu XD, Li MY. Accuracy of whole-body PET and PET-CT in initial M staging of head and neck cancer: a meta-analysis. Head Neck. 2011;33(1):87–94.
11. Xu G, Li J, Zuo X, Li C. Comparison of whole body positron emission tomography (PET)/PET-computed tomography and conventional anatomic imaging for detecting distant malignancies in patients with head and neck cancer: a meta-analysis. Laryngoscope. 2012;122(9):1974–8.
12. Arias F, Chicata V, Garcia-Velloso MJ, Asin G, Uzcanga M, Eito C, et al. Impact of initial FDG PET/CT in the management plan of patients with locally advanced head and neck cancer. Clin Transl Oncol. 2015;17(2):139–44.
13. Yongkui L, Jian L, Wanghan, Jingui L. 18FDG-PET/CT for the detection of regional nodal metastasis in patients with primary head and neck cancer before treatment: a meta-analysis. Surg Oncol. 2013;22(2):e11–6.
14. Kyzas PA, Evangelou E, Denaxa-Kyza D, Ioannidis JP. 18F-fluorodeoxyglucose positron emission tomography to evaluate cervical node metastases in patients with head and neck squamous cell carcinoma: a meta-analysis. J Natl Cancer Inst. 2008;100(10):712–20.
15. Nakamoto Y, Tatsumi M, Hammoud D, Cohade C, Osman MM, Wahl RL. Normal FDG distribution patterns in the head and neck: PET/CT evaluation. Radiology. 2005;234(3):879–85.
16. Hojgaard L, Berthelsen AK, Loft A. Head and neck: normal variations and benign findings in FDG positron emission tomography/computed tomography imaging. PET clinics. 2014;9(2):141–5.
17. Blodgett TM, Fukui MB, Snyderman CH, Branstetter BFT, McCook BM, Townsend DW, et al. Combined PET-CT in the head and neck: part 1. Physiologic, altered physiologic, and artifactual FDG uptake. Radiographics. 2005;25(4):897–912.
18. Loevner LA, Kim AK, Mikityansky I. PET/CT-MR imaging in head and neck cancer including pitfalls and physiologic variations. PET clinics. 2008;3(3):335–53.
19. Wedman J, Pruim J, Roodenburg JL, Halmos GB, Langedijk JA, Dierckx RA, et al. Alternative PET tracers in head and neck cancer. A review. Eur Arch Otorhinolaryngol. 2013;270(10):2595–601.
20. Heuveling DA, de Bree R, van Dongen GA. The potential role of non-FDG-PET in the management of head and neck cancer. Oral Oncol. 2011;47(1):2–7.
21. Woods C, Sohn J, Yao M. The application of PET in radiation treatment planning for head and neck cancer. PET clinics. 2011;6(2):149–63.
22. Awan MJ, Siddiqui F, Schwartz D, Yuan J, Machtay M, Yao M. Application of positron emission tomography/computed tomography in radiation treatment planning for head and neck cancers. World J Radiol. 2015;7(11):382–93.

23. Delouya G, Igidbashian L, Houle A, Belair M, Boucher L, Cohade C, et al. (1)(8)F-FDG-PET imaging in radiotherapy tumor volume delineation in treatment of head and neck cancer. Radiother Oncol. 2011;101(3):362–8.
24. Gill BS, Pai SS, McKenzie S, Beriwal S. Utility of PET for radiotherapy treatment planning. PET clinics. 2015;10(4):541–54.
25. Annunziata S, Caldarella C, Treglia G. Cost-effectiveness of fluorine-18-fluorodeoxyglucose positron emission tomography in tumours other than lung cancer: a systematic review. World J Radiol. 2014;6(3):48–55.
26. Smith AF, Hall PS, Hulme CT, Dunn JA, McConkey CC, Rahman JK, et al. Cost-effectiveness analysis of PET-CT-guided management for locally advanced head and neck cancer. Eur J Cancer. 2017;85:6–14.

Lymphoma

19

1. What are the types of lymphoma?

   There are two subtypes, Hodgkin lymphoma (HL) and non-Hodgkin lymphoma (NHL). NHL is further divided into B-cell and T-cell lymphomas.

2. What is the percentage of fluorodeoxyglucose (FDG) avidity in various subtypes of lymphomas?

   FDG avidity of various subtypes of lymphomas is as follows:

   HL (97–100%)
   Diffuse large B cell lymphoma (DLBCL—97–100%)
   Follicular lymphoma (FL—91–100%)
   Mantle-cell lymphoma (100%)
   Burkitt's lymphoma (100%)
   Marginal zone lymphoma, nodal (100%)
   Lymphoblastic lymphoma (100%)
   Anaplastic large T-cell lymphoma (94–100%),
   NK/T-cell lymphoma (83–100%)
   Angioimmunoblastic T-cell lymphoma (78–100%)
   Peripheral T-cell lymphoma (86–98%)
   MALT marginal zone lymphoma (54–81%)
   Small lymphocytic lymphoma (47–83%)
   Enteropathy-type T-cell lymphoma (67–100%)
   Splenic marginal zone lymphoma (53–67%)
   Mycosis fungoides (83–100%)
   Sezary syndrome (100%)
   Primary cutaneous anaplastic large T-cell lymphoma (40–60%)
   Lymphomatoid papulosis (50%)
   Subcutaneous panniculitis-like T-cell lymphoma (71%)
   Cutaneous B-cell lymphoma (0%) [1–3]

© The Author(s), under exclusive license to Springer Nature Switzerland AG 2026
S. Raja et al., *Question and Answers in PET/CT*,
https://doi.org/10.1007/978-3-032-00821-3_19

3. What is the role of 18F-FDG positron emission tomography (PET)-computed tomography (CT) in HL?

   18F-FDG PET-CT has an established role in staging and end-of-treatment (EoT) response evaluation of HL. There is evidence of a role in interim treatment assessment of HL for adapted therapy. However, its implications are yet to be proven. 18F-FDG PET-CT also excludes the need for routine bone marrow biopsies as it accurately identifies the marrow involvement [4–6].

4. What is the role of 18F-FDG PET-CT in diagnosing HL?

   Diagnosing lymphoma requires assessment of histopathological morphology, immunohistochemistry, and flow cytometry, as well as, where appropriate, molecular studies to categorize the lymphoma accurately. 18F-FDG PET-CT does not help diagnose HL, as there are hypermetabolic mimics such as tuberculosis, sarcoidosis, metastatic disease, and so on. However, FDG PET-CT can guide biopsy targets [1, 6].

5. What is the role of 18F-FDG PET-CT in staging HL?

   18F-FDG PET-CT is highly sensitive in detecting nodal and extranodal (including spleen and bone marrow) disease in HL compared to CT. 18F-FDG PET-CT consistently influences staging, with upstaging in approximately 15–25% of patients and downstaging in only a small number [4].

6. What is the role of 18F-FDG PET-CT in the assessment of treatment response in HL?

   18F-FDG PET-CT is the standard of care in EoT assessment of early- and advanced-stage HL with a negative predictive value of 95–100% and a positive predictive value of more than 90%.

   Interim 18F-FDG PET-CT is superior to CT in assessing early response and providing prognostic information—progression-free survival and overall survival. Various trials are evaluating the role of PET response-adapted therapy; however, currently, it is not recommended to change the treatment solely based on interim PET-CT unless there is clear evidence of progression [1, 5, 7].

7. What is the role of 18F-FDG PET-CT in the surveillance of HL?

   18F-FDG-PET/CT is not routinely recommended for surveillance of HL patients because of its low positive predictive value, additional radiation exposure, and uncertainty on the impact on overall survival. However, 18F-FDG PET/CT is preferable in restaging if there is clinical suspicion of relapse, as it has been shown to be more accurate than CT [8].

8. What are the sensitivity and specificity of 18F-FDG PET/CT in the assessment of HL?

   The sensitivity and specificity of 18F-FDG PET-CT in detecting HL are more than 95% [9, 10].

9. What are the common pitfalls of 18F-FDG PET-CT in staging HL?

   Sites of high physiological FDG uptake, such as the brain, myocardium, gastrointestinal tract, urinary tract, lymphoid tissue, brown adipose tissue, salivary glands, and thymus, may obscure or mimic the presence of disease. Benign conditions with increased glycolysis, such as infection, inflammation, and granulomatous disease, may also increase FDG uptake [10].

10. What are the common false-positive 18F-FDG PET-CT findings in HL?

Common false-positive 18F-FDG PET-CT findings in HL include the following:

(a) Physiological tracer uptake in brown fat, Waldeyer's ring, muscles, and thymus
(b) Active infective/inflammatory conditions like tuberculosis or sarcoidosis, and so on
(c) Reactive bone marrow uptake (usually diffuse uptake)
(d) Treatment-related changes such as bleomycin-induced lung changes, radiotherapy (RT)-induced inflammation, thymic rebound hyperplasia, diffuse bone marrow/splenic uptake following colony-stimulating factors, and so on
(e) FDG uptake by (non-neoplastic) microenvironment cells such as CD8+ tumor-infiltrating lymphocytes and PD1-positive lymphocytes within the tumor
(f) In addition, various artifacts such as misregistration artifact, partial volume effect, attenuation correction artifact, and truncation artifact can result in false positives, and so on [7, 10, 11].

11. What are the common false-negative 18F-FDG PET-CT findings in Hodgkin's lymphoma?

The common false-negative 18F-FDG PET-CT findings in HL include the following:

(a) Small-sized lesions/lymph nodes (smaller than the resolution of the PET scanner)
(b) A very small percentage (<3%) of HL can have little or no FDG avidity
(c) Post-chemotherapy status
(d) Artifacts such as misregistration artifacts, and so on [10–12]

12. What is the cost-effectiveness of 18F-FDG PET-CT in HL management?

18F-FDG PET-CT is more accurate than CT and bone marrow biopsy (BMB) in HL staging and restaging. There is limited data on the cost-effectiveness of 18F-FDG PET-CT in the management of HL, but overall, 18F-FDG PET-CT is highly cost-effective [13, 14].

13. What are the advantages and limitations of FDG PET-CT in HL?

Advantages: 18F-FDG PET-CT is the standard of care in staging and EoT response evaluation of HL. It is helpful in the interim treatment assessment of HL and provides prognostic information. 18F-FDG PET-CT also excludes the need for routine bone marrow biopsies, as it identifies the marrow involvement accurately.

Limitations: The interim PET response-adapted therapy concept is yet to be validated. It is not recommended for routine surveillance of HL [4–6, 8].

14. What is the Deauville five-point scale (5-PS)?

Deauville 5-PS is a response evaluation criterion used for interim and EoT response evaluation of FDG-avid lymphomas (HL, DLBCL, and FL).

The 5-PS scores the most intense uptake in a site of initial disease, if present, as follows:

1. No uptake
2. Uptake ≤ mediastinum
3. Uptake > mediastinum but ≤ liver
4. Uptake moderately higher than liver
5. Uptake markedly higher than liver and/or new lesions
   X. New areas of uptake unlikely to be related to lymphoma [1, 15]

15. What is complete metabolic response (CMR)?

CMR is the visual or quantitative measure of the overall success of treatment. It is a powerful positive prognostic indicator. A Deauville score of 1 or 2 is considered to represent a CMR at the interim and end of treatment. Sometimes, particularly in research, a Deauville score of 3 is regarded as a CMR. However, in response-adapted trials exploring treatment de-escalation, a more cautious approach may be preferred, judging a score of 3 to be an inadequate response to avoid undertreatment. Therefore, the interpretation of a score of 3 depends on the timing of the assessment, the clinical context, and the treatment [6].

16. What is the role of 18F-FDG PET-CT in NHL?

18F-FDG PET-CT is indicated in staging and EoT evaluation of all FDG-avid NHL. Its use in interim treatment response assessment is yet to be validated. It is not routinely recommended for surveillance follow-up of NHL. 18F-FDG PET-CT is not useful in evaluating less/non-FDG avid NHL (such as Chronic Lymphocytic Leukemia/Small Lymphocytic Lymphoma (CLL/SLL), Mucosa-Associated Lymphoid Tissue (MALT)/splenic marginal zone lymphoma, cutaneous T cell lymphomas including mycosis fungoides). [4, 5, 7, 8]

17. What is the role of 18F-FDG PET-CT in the diagnosis of NHL?

Diagnosing lymphoma requires assessment of histological morphology, immunohistochemistry, and flow cytometry, as well as, where appropriate, molecular studies to categorize the lymphoma accurately. 18F-FDG PET-CT is not useful in diagnosing HL, as there are hypermetabolic mimics such as tuberculosis, sarcoidosis, metastatic disease, and so on. However, FDG PET-CT can guide biopsy targets [1, 6].

18. What is the role of 18F-FDG PET-CT in staging NHL?

18F-FDG PET-CT is the standard of care in staging all FDG-avid aggressive NHL, such as DLBCL, mantle cell lymphoma, and peripheral T cell lymphoma (PTCL).

However, 18F-FDG PET-CT may be considered in staging indolent NHL (such as follicular lymphomas) and extranodal lymphomas because it may lead to a change in a clinical stage in some patients and guide the choice of follow-up imaging modality. Another role is the workup of suspected transformation to a higher-grade lymphoma (Richter transformation) in lymphomas such as FL, CLL/SLL, and marginal zone lymphoma [4, 8].

19. What is the role of 18F-FDG PET-CT in the assessment of treatment response in NHLs?

    The Lugano classification recommends 18F-FDG PET-CT for EoT DLBCL and Follicular lymphoma assessment. Although 18F-FDG PET-CT may be considered for the EoT evaluation of other aggressive NHL-like mantle cells and aggressive peripheral T-cell lymphomas, the lack of effective treatment regimens for durable remission renders an uncertain role for FDG PET-CT in response evaluation. Despite its high NPV of greater than 80%, the role of interim 18F-FDG PET-CT in NHL is limited because of the low PPV (as low as 15%) [5, 7, 8, 16, 17].

20. What is the role of 18F-FDG PET-CT in the surveillance of NHL?

    18F-FDG-PET/CT is not routinely recommended for surveillance follow-up of NHL patients because of its low positive predictive value, additional radiation exposure, and uncertainty on the impact on overall survival. However, 18F-FDG PET/CT is preferable in restaging if there is clinical suspicion of relapse, as the technique appears more accurate than CT [8].

21. What is the role of 18F-FDG PET-CT in low-grade lymphomas?

    18F-FDG PET-CT is useful in staging FDG-avid low-grade NHL, such as follicular lymphoma, nodal marginal zone lymphoma, and so on, because it may lead to a change in clinical stage in some patients and guide the choice of follow-up imaging modality. An additional role is the workup of suspected transformation to a higher-grade lymphoma and guiding site for confirmatory biopsy [4, 8].

22. What is the role of 18F-FDG PET-CT in mycosis fungoides?

    18F-FDG PET-CT is not useful in primary T cell cutaneous lymphomas, including mycosis fungoides, as they are usually FDG less/non-avid [4, 8].

23. What are the common pitfalls of 18F-FDG PET-CT in staging NHL?

    Sites of high physiological uptake, such as the brain, myocardium, gastrointestinal tract, urinary tract, lymphoid tissue, brown adipose tissue, salivary glands, and thymus, may obscure or mimic the presence of disease. Benign conditions with increased glycolysis, such as infection, inflammation, and granulomatous disease, may also increase FDG uptake. A few low-grade NHLs can be non-FDG avid [10].

24. What are the common false-positive 18F-FDG PET-CT findings in NHL?

The common false-positive 18F-FDG PET-CT findings in NHL include the following:

(a) Physiological tracer uptake in brown fat, Waldeyer's ring, muscles, and thymus
(b) Active infective/inflammatory conditions like tuberculosis or sarcoidosis, and so on
(c) Reactive bone marrow uptake (usually low-grade diffuse uptake)
(d) Treatment-related changes such as chemotherapy-induced lung changes, RT-induced inflammation, thymic rebound hyperplasia, diffuse bone marrow/splenic uptake following colony-stimulating factors, and so on
(e) FDG uptake by (non-neoplastic) microenvironment cells such as CD8+ tumor-infiltrating lymphocytes and PD1-positive lymphocytes in the tumor
(f) In addition, various artifacts such as misregistration artifact, partial volume effect, attenuation correction artifact, and truncation artifact can result in false positives, and so on [7, 10, 11].

25. What are the common false-negative 18F-FDG PET-CT findings in NHL?

The common false-negative 18F-FDG PET-CT findings in NHL include the following:

(a) FDG non/less avid lymphomas such as CLL/SLL, splenic/extranodal marginal zone lymphoma, mycosis fungoides, and so on
(b) Small-sized lesions/lymph nodes (smaller than the resolution of the PET scanner)
(c) Post-chemotherapy status
(d) Artifacts like misregistration artifacts, and so on [10–12]

26. What is the cost-effectiveness of 18F-FDG PET-CT in NHL management?

18F-FDG PET-CT is accurate and cost-effective in the initial staging of NHL. Routine use of imaging, including 18F-FDG PET-CT, is not cost-effective in the surveillance of NHL [18, 19].

27. What are the advantages and limitations of 18F-FDG PET-CT in NHL?

Advantages: 18F-FDG PET-CT is useful in staging all FDG-avid NHL and in the EoT response evaluation of DLBCL and FL. 18F-FDG PET-CT also excludes the need for routine bone marrow biopsies in most patients with DLBCL.

Limitations: 18F-FDG PET-CT is not useful in FDG less/non-avid NHL. The PPV of interim PET in the NHL is very poor. It is not routinely recommended for surveillance of the NHL [1, 4–6, 8].

28. What is the role of 18F-FDG PET-CT in the assessment of bone marrow disease?

Focal bone marrow FDG uptake is considered positive for bone marrow involvement by lymphoma. Interpretation of diffuse bone marrow FDG uptake may vary according to lymphoma subtype because BMB positivity is rare in HL patients with diffuse uptake. In contrast, positive BMB has been reported in many DLBCL patients with diffuse uptake.

Nevertheless, several studies have shown that the sensitivity of bone marrow assessment in 18F-FDG PET/CT is higher than BMB in HL and DLBCL. Thus, routine BMB (which was considered the gold standard for detecting bone marrow infiltration) is no longer deemed essential to HL, and in most patients with DLBCL, unless in the latter, that 18F-FDG PET/CT was negative, and it was necessary to determine if discordant histology was present in the bone marrow. The sensitivity of 18F-FDG PET-CT is low in detecting bone marrow involvement in other lymphomas, such as FL and PTCL, where BMB is recommended if the detection of bone marrow involvement would impact the treatment strategy [4, 20–23].

29. What is the role of 18F-FDG PET-CT in guiding invasive procedures?

For patients in whom discordant histology is suspected, 18F-FDG PET-CT is useful in identifying the optimal site for confirmatory biopsy. Despite its high negative predictive value at the end of therapy response assessment, 18F-FDG PET/CT has a relatively low positive predictive value, thereby warranting biopsy of residual metabolically active tissue in patients with lymphoma before any salvage therapy is planned. 18F-FDG PET/CT plays a role in directing biopsy target(s) in patients with indolent NHL suspected of transformation into aggressive disease [6, 8, 12].

30. What is the relationship between the intensity of FDG uptake and lymphoma grade?

In general, the intensity of FDG uptake is directly proportional to the lymphoma grade. Low-grade lymphomas accumulate less FDG, while higher-grade lymphomas accumulate more FDG [24, 25].

31. What is the ideal time to image after chemotherapy and RT?

18F-FDG PET-CT should ideally be performed 3 weeks after the chemotherapy. Suppose an interim PET is planned, and the next cycle of chemotherapy is due within 2 weeks. In that case, it should not be performed earlier than 14 days after the last chemotherapy cycle because therapy's "stunning" effect on tumor cells exists for up to 10 days and therapy-induced inflammatory FDG uptake may persist for up to 13–14 days. 18F-FDG PET-CT should ideally be performed 3 months following completion of RT; however, PET/CT can also be performed after 6–8 weeks of RT if early assessment is required clinically [1, 26, 27].

32. What is the role of 18F-FDG PET-CT in RT planning of lymphoma?

Since 18F-FDG PET-CT is the modality of choice for optimal staging of most types of lymphomas, many studies have shown that it impacts the gross tumor volume (GTV) in the majority of patients with lymphoma compared to CT-based planning by either increasing or decreasing the GTV, as well as excluding or including RT in some patients by upstaging/downstaging disease. Overall, 18F-FDG PET/CT can contribute to achieving the highest chance of cure with the least long-term side effects [28–30].

Acquiring PET/CT in RT treatment position on a flat tabletop with appropriate immobilization devices, skin markers, and respiratory gating (where required) potentially avoids difficulties in contouring during RT treatment planning as well as minimizes lesion FDG inhomogeneity secondary to motion artifacts [31].

33. What is the utility of 18F-FDG PET-CT in stem cell transplantation?

High-dose chemotherapy and autologous stem cell transplantation (ASCT) can offer durable remission in many patients with relapsed or high-risk lymphoma. Many studies have shown that 18F-FDG PET/CT is superior to conventional CT for determining the chemosensitivity of lymphoma, which is an essential parameter in predicting outcomes following ASCT. PFS and OS are significantly higher in chemosensitive patients (i.e., Deauville 1–3). Thus, FDG PET/CT is recommended in patients with relapsed/refractory HL or DLBCL after salvage chemotherapy to guide decisions before high-dose chemotherapy and ASCT. However, a recent meta-analysis revealed only a moderate predictive value for NHL compared to a high predictive value for HL, which was attributed mainly to the poor quality of included studies in the NHL group [1, 8, 32–35].

34. What is the role of 18F-FDG PET/CT in immunotherapy response assessment?

Immunotherapy (e.g., PD-L1 checkpoint inhibitors) has shown promising results in the treatment of refractory and relapsed lymphoma. Reporters should be aware of potential delayed and flare responses, where lesions increase in size, and FDG avidity and new lesions appear but later resolve/remain stable. Lymphoma response to immunomodulatory therapy criteria has been introduced for 18F-FDG PET/CT evaluation of lymphoma following immunotherapy [36].

- IR 1: ≥50% increase in the sum of the product of the perpendicular diameters (SPD) of up to six target measurable nodes and extranodal sites occurred in the first 12 weeks of therapy and without clinical deterioration
- IR 2: new lesions or ≥50% increase of existing lesion(s) without a ≥50% increase of overall tumor burden at any time during treatment
- IR 3: increased FDG uptake of one or more lesions without any increase in size or number of those lesions.

In the event of indeterminate response (IR), biopsy or repeated imaging within 12 weeks is suggested to confirm true progressive disease versus flare or pseudo-progression.

Preliminary data suggests that the incidence of pseudoprogression may be lower in lymphoma than in solid tumors. In addition, early FDG PET/CT assessment in HL predicted OS and allowed early risk stratification [37].

Immune-related side adverse events can involve a variety of organs and may be evident on 18F-FDG PET/CT. These include thyroiditis, colitis, pneumonitis, arthritis, and pancreatitis [36].

References

1. Barrington SF, Mikhaeel NG, Kostakoglu L, et al. Role of imaging in the staging and response assessment of lymphoma: consensus of the international conference on malignant lymphomas imaging working group. J Clin Oncol. 2014;32(27):3048–58.
2. Elstrom R, Guan L, Baker G, et al. Utility of FDG-PET scanning in lymphoma by WHO classification. Blood. 2003;101:3875–6.
3. Weiler-Sagie M, Bushelev O, Epelbaum R, et al. (18)F-FDG avidity in lymphoma readdressed: a study of 766 patients. J Nucl Med. 2010;51:25–30.
4. El-Galaly TC, Gormsen LC, Hutchings M. PET/CT for staging; past, present, and future. Semin Nucl Med. 2018;48(1):4–16.
5. Kobe C, Dietlein M, Hellwig D. PET/CT for lymphoma post-therapy response assessment in Hodgkin lymphoma and diffuse large B-cell lymphoma. Semin Nucl Med. 2018;48(1):28–36.
6. Cheson BD, Fisher RI, Barrington SF, et al. Recommendations for initial evaluation, staging, and response assessment of Hodgkin and non-Hodgkin lymphoma: the Lugano classification. J Clin Oncol. 2014;32(27):3059–68.
7. Gallamini A, Zwarthoed C. Interim FDG-PET imaging in lymphoma. Semin Nucl Med. 2018;48(1):17–27.
8. Karls S, Shah H, Jacene H. PET/CT for lymphoma post-therapy response assessment in other lymphomas, response assessment for autologous stem cell transplant, and lymphoma follow-up. Semin Nucl Med. 2018;48(1):37–49.
9. Kabickova E, Sumerauer D, Cumlivska E, et al. Comparison of 18F-FDG-PET and standard procedures for the pretreatment staging of children and adolescents with Hodgkin's disease. Eur J Nucl Med Mol Imaging. 2006;33:1025–31.
10. D'souza MM, Jaimini A, Bansal A, et al. FDG-PET/CT in lymphoma. Indian J Radiol Imaging. 2013;23(4):354–65.
11. Corrigan AJ, Schleyer PJ, Cook GJ. Pitfalls and artifacts in the use of PET/CT in oncology imaging. Semin Nucl Med. 2015;45(6):481–99.
12. Subocz E, Hałka J, Dziuk M. The role of FDG-PET in Hodgkin lymphoma. Contemp Oncol (Pozn). 2017;21(2):104–14.
13. Cerci JJ, Trindade E, Buccheri V, et al. Consistency of FDG-PET accuracy and cost-effectiveness in initial staging of patients with Hodgkin lymphoma across jurisdictions. Clin Lymphoma Myeloma Leuk. 2011;11(4):314–20.
14. Cerci JJ, Trindade E, Pracchia LF, et al. Cost effectiveness of positron emission tomography in patients with Hodgkin's lymphoma in unconfirmed complete remission or partial remission after first-line therapy. J Clin Oncol. 2010;28(8):1415–21.
15. Meignan M, Gallamini A, Haioun C. Report on the first international workshop on interim-PETScan in lymphoma. Leuk Lymphoma. 2009;50:1257–60.
16. Adams HJA, Kwee TC. Interim FDG-PET in lymphoma, a questionable practice in hematology. Eur J Nucl Med Mol Imaging. 2017;44(12):2014–7.
17. Lazarovici J, Terroir M, Arfi-Rouche J, et al. Poor predictive value of positive interim FDG-PET/CT in primary mediastinal large B-cell lymphoma. Eur J Nucl Med Mol Imaging. 2017;44(12):2018–24.
18. Klose T, Leidl R, Buchmann I, Brambs HJ, Reske SN. Primary staging of lymphomas: cost-effectiveness of FDG-PET versus computed tomography. Eur J Nucl Med. 2000;27(10):1457–64.
19. Huntington SF, Svoboda J, Doshi JA. Cost-effectiveness analysis of routine surveillance imaging of patients with diffuse large B-cell lymphoma in first remission. J Clin Oncol. 2015;33(13):1467–74.
20. Cheson BD. PET/CT in lymphoma: current overview and future directions. Semin Nucl Med. 2018;48(1):76–81.

21. El-Galaly TC, D'Amore F, Mylam KJ, et al. Routine bone marrow biopsy has little or no therapeutic consequence for PET/CT staged treatment naive Hodgkin lymphoma patients. J Clin Oncol. 2012;30:4508–14.
22. Khan AB, Barrington SF, Mikhaeel G, et al. PET-CT staging of DLBCL accurately identifies and provides new insights into the clinical significance of bone marrow involvement. Blood. 2013;122:61–7.
23. Chen-Liang TH, Martin-Santos T, Jerez A, et al. The role of bone marrow biopsy and FDG-PET/CT in identifying bone marrow infiltration in the initial diagnosis of high grade non-Hodgkin B-cell lymphoma and Hodgkin lymphoma. Accuracy in a multicenter series of 372 patients. Am J Hematol. 2015;90:686–90.
24. Rodriguez M, Rehn S, Ahlstrom H, et al. Predicting malignancy grade with PET in non-Hodgkin's lymphoma. J Nucl Med. 1995;36:1790–6.
25. Schoder H, Noy A, Gonen M, et al. Intensity of 18fluorodeoxyglucose uptake in positron emission tomography distinguishes between indolent and aggressive non-Hodgkin's lymphoma. J Clin Oncol. 2005;23:4643–51.
26. Boellaard R, O'Doherty MJ, Weber WA, et al. FDG PET and PET/CT: EANM procedure guidelines for tumour PET imaging—version 1.0. Eur J Nucl Med Mol Imaging. 2010;37:181–200.
27. Surasi DS, Bhambhvani P, Baldwin JA, Almodovar SE, O'Malley JP. 18F-FDG PET and PET/CT patient preparation: a review of the literature. J Nucl Med Technol. 2014;42(1):5–13.
28. Girinsky T, Auperin A, Ribrag V, et al. Role of FDG-PET in the implementation of involved-node radiation therapy for Hodgkin lymphoma patients. Int J Radiat Oncol Biol Phys. 2014;89:1047–52.
29. Terezakis SA, Schoder H, Kowalski A, et al. A prospective study of (1)(8)FDG-PET with CT coregistration for radiation treatment planning of lymphomas and other hematologic malignancies. Int J Radiat Oncol Biol Phys. 2014;89:376–83.
30. Bird D, Patel C, Scarsbrook AF, et al. Evaluation of clinical target volume expansion required for involved site neck radiotherapy for lymphoma to account for the absence of a pre-chemotherapy PET-CT in the radiotherapy treatment position. Radiother Oncol. 2017;124:161–7.
31. Specht L, Berthelsen AK. PET/CT in radiation therapy planning. Semin Nucl Med. 2017;48:67–75.
32. Qiao W, Zhao J, Wang C, et al. Predictive value of (18)F-FDG hybrid PET/CT for the clinical outcome in patients with non-Hodgkin's lymphoma prior to and after autologous stem cell transplantation. Hematology. 2010;15:21–7.
33. Moskowitz CH, Matasar MJ, Zelenetz AD, et al. Normalization of pre-ASCT, FDG-PET imaging with second-line, non-cross-resistant, chemotherapy programs improves event-free survival in patients with Hodgkin lymphoma. Blood. 2012;119:1665–70.
34. Adams HJ, Kwee TC. Pretransplant FDG-PET in aggressive nonHodgkin lymphoma: systematic review and meta-analysis. Eur J Haematol. 2017;98:337–47.
35. Adams HJ, Kwee TC. Prognostic value of pretransplant FDG-PET in refractory/relapsed Hodgkin lymphoma treated with autologous stem cell transplantation: systematic review and meta-analysis. Ann Hematol. 2016;95:695–706.
36. Barrington SF, Johnson PWM. 18F-FDG PET/CT in lymphoma: has imaging-directed personalized medicine become a reality? J Nucl Med. 2017;58(10):1539–44.
37. Chen A, Mokrane FZ, Schwartz LH, et al. Early 18F-FDG PET/CT response predicts survival in relapsed or refractory Hodgkin lymphoma treated with Nivolumab. J Nucl Med. 2020;61:649–54.

Esophageal Cancer

1. What are the histological subtypes of esophageal cancer?

    Over 90% of esophageal carcinomas are squamous cell carcinoma (SCC) or adenocarcinoma. SCC is often found in the upper and middle third of the esophagus, whereas adenocarcinoma occurs in the lower esophagus. Other rare types include adenosquamous carcinoma, small cell carcinoma, undifferentiated carcinoma, carcinoid tumor, gastrointestinal stromal tumor, leiomyosarcoma, rhabdomyosarcoma, Kaposi sarcoma, malignant melanoma, and lymphoma [1].

2. What are the common indications of ^{18}F-fluorodeoxyglucose (18F-FDG) positron emission tomography (PET)/computed tomography (CT) in esophageal cancer?
    (a) Initial staging
    (b) Response assessment after neoadjuvant therapy
    (c) Palliative therapy
    (d) Detection of disease recurrence and restaging
    (e) Radiotherapy planning
    (f) Predicting prognosis [1–3]

3. What is the role of 18F-FDG PET and PET/CT in diagnosing esophageal cancer?
    18F-FDG PET/CT is not routinely recommended in the diagnosis of esophageal cancer or as a screening test [1].

4. What is the role of 18F-FDG PET/CT in staging esophageal cancer?

    CT and/or endoscopic ultrasound (EUS) are preferred for initial tumor T and N staging. EUS enables a more accurate measurement of the depth of invasion [4]. However, FDG PET/CT is useful in detecting tumor involvement in normal-sized lymph nodes, remote lymph nodal, and distant metastases [5]. The most common sites of distant metastases are the lungs, liver, and distant lymph nodes.

With Contributions by Dr. Arun Visakh R

S. Raja et al., *Question and Answers in PET/CT*,
https://doi.org/10.1007/978-3-032-00821-3_20

5. What is the role of 18F-FDG PET/CT in the assessment of treatment response in esophageal cancer?

PET/CT is useful in evaluating the response to neoadjuvant chemotherapy and radiotherapy by distinguishing residual viable tumor from fibrosis/necrosis based on the metabolic activity of the tumor [6], thereby providing a functional alternative to the anatomical assessment. Identifying non-responders early during treatment can help appropriately select patients for surgery, thus avoiding the toxic side effects of therapy [7, 8]. To avoid false-positive results due to treatment-related inflammation, post-treatment FDG PET/CT should be performed 3 weeks after completion of radiotherapy. 18F-FDG PET and PET/CT are valuable for predicting response [14].

6. What is the role of 18F-FDG PET/CT in restaging esophageal cancer following definitive surgery?

PET/CT scanning is often used to detect recurrent or metastatic disease after esophagectomy [9, 10]. Local disease recurrence near the anastomotic site, which may be a subtle finding on diagnostic CT scans alone, can be better detected by PET scans. It is particularly useful in detecting new interval metastases that are either occult or difficult to diagnose prospectively on conventional imaging and is, therefore, useful in the follow-up of esophageal malignancy [11].

7. What is the sensitivity of 18F-FDG PET/CT in the assessment of the primary esophageal tumor?

Among primary tumors, 68–100% show FDG uptake, whereas early-stage T1 and T2 tumors tend to have minimal or no FDG uptake, likely secondary to a lower degree of cellular proliferation in these smaller tumors [1, 12, 13]. Most false negatives in SCC are due to small-volume tumors, whereas non-avid adenocarcinomas are often poorly differentiated, showing diffuse nonintentional growth and mucus-containing tumor types [14].

8. What are the sensitivity and specificity of 18F-FDG PET/CT in the assessment of distant metastasis?

The sensitivity and specificity of 18F-FDG PET/CT in detecting metastatic disease are 79% and 95%, respectively [15]. FDG PET/CT scanning has been shown to provide improved staging information and change in management in about one-third of patients, compared with EUS and CT imaging [1, 16]. The limiting factor to distant metastasis detection sensitivity is the lesion size, with an approximate minimum threshold of 1 cm [17].

9. What is the role of 18F-FDG PET/CT in T and N staging?

EUS is superior to FDG PET/CT for accurate T staging of primary tumors [18]. However, FDG PET/CT may play a complementary role to EUS for the assessment of T4b disease. The sensitivity of 18F-FDG PET/CT in detecting locoregional lymph node metastases is poor (55%) because of the high scattered activity around FDG-avid primary tumors, where EUS is considered superior. However, it is highly accurate (around 90%) in detecting remote lymph nodal metastases [4].

10. What is the role of 18F-FDG PET and PET/CT in M staging?

The main role of FDG PET/CT scanning in the initial staging of esophageal cancer lies in its superior ability to detect stage IV disease. FDG PET/CT scanning is preferred, if there is no evidence of distant metastatic disease in conventional imaging. This is important in avoiding unnecessary or ineffective surgical intervention in cases with occult metastases [19].

11. What are the common pitfalls of 18F-FDG PET/CT in esophageal cancer?

The common pitfalls of 18F-FDG PET-CT in esophageal cancer include the following:

(a) Physiological/ inflammatory esophageal FDG uptake
(b) Technical artifacts due to misregistration, partial volume effect, attenuation correction, and truncation effect
(c) Reduced spatial and contrast resolutions of PET/CT limit evaluation of the depth of local tumor invasion and detection of metastatic dissemination to locoregional lymph nodes that are anatomically close to the primary tumor
(d) Treatment-related pitfalls are due to surgery, chemotherapy, and radiotherapy [20, 21].

12. What are the common false-positive findings of 18F-FDG PET/CT in esophageal cancer?

The common false-positive findings include infection/inflammatory conditions, surgical treatment-related changes, post-radiotherapy inflammation, chemotherapy-induced lung changes, and so on. Mild, focal uptake at the gastroesophageal junction is frequently identified. In addition, various artifacts such as misregistration artifacts, partial volume effect, attenuation correction artifacts, and truncation artifacts can result in false positives [22].

13. What are the common false-negative findings of 18F-FDG PET/CT in esophageal cancer?

The common false-negative 18F-FDG PET/CT findings in colorectal cancer are as follows:

1. Small-sized lesions/lymph nodes beyond the resolution of the PET scanner
2. Post-chemotherapy status
3. Artifacts like misregistration artifact and so on (20%)

14. What are the non-FDG tracers in imaging esophageal cancer?
(a) Hypoxia agents—for example, F-18 fluoromisonidasole
(b) Proliferative marker—for example, F-18 fluorothymidine [23]

15. What is the role of 18F-FDG PET/CT in the management of esophageal cancer?
(a) In the initial evaluation of esophageal cancer, FDG PET/CT has a superior ability to detect stage IV disease [19].
(b) Early response assessment with FDG-PET/CT distinguishes responders from non-responders and can help to appropriately select patients for surgery, thus avoiding the toxic side effects of therapy [7, 8].

(c) PET/CT scanning is often used to detect recurrent or metastatic disease after esophagectomy [9, 10].

(d) FDG PET/CT is useful in radiotherapy planning of esophageal cancers.

16. What is the role of 18F-FDG PET-CT in radiotherapy planning in esophageal cancer?

   The addition of 18F-FDG PET to the planning CT in radiotherapy significantly impacts target volume delineation (in 20–94% of patients), resulting in either a reduction or an increase in tumor volumes based on CT images [12].

17. What are the limitations of 18F-FDG PET/CT in radiotherapy planning?

   (a) The relatively lower sensitivity for the primary tumor means the irradiated volume should not be based on the negativity of FDG avidity if malignant involvement is suspected on other imaging investigations [24].

   (b) Inability to differentiate FDG avidity between *in vivo* tumor and inflammation.

   (c) Several methods (percentage of maximum SUV, fixed SUV cut off of 2.5, and confidence-connected region-growing method) have been described for tumor volume segmentation. However, the optimal method for tumor volume segmentation is yet to be standardized and validated [12].

18. What are the advantages and limitations of 18F-FDG PET/CT in esophageal cancer?

Advantages:

1. Very useful in the assessment of distant metastases.
2. Response assessment following neoadjuvant chemotherapy and radiotherapy by distinguishing residual viable tumor from fibrosis/necrosis based on the metabolic activity of the tumor [6].
3. Identification of non-responders early during treatment can help to appropriately select patients for surgery, thus avoiding the toxic side effects of therapy.
4. PET/CT is widely adopted to evaluate recurrent or metastatic disease after esophagectomy [9, 10].
5. The addition of FDG-PET in radiotherapy planning has a significant impact on target volume delineation [12].

Limitations:

1. FDG avidity is low in a few tumor subtypes (e.g., poorly differentiated tumors, non-intestinal growth type, and mucus-containing tumors) and small-sized lesions/lymph nodes
2. Non-specific nature of the tracer with various false-positive findings
3. Lack of standardization of methods used for tumor volume segmentation in radiotherapy planning
4. Relatively high cost and radiation exposure [1, 22]

References

1. Kwee RM, Marcus C, Sheikhbahaei S, Subramaniam RM. PET with Fluorodeoxyglucose F 18/computed tomography in the clinical management and patient outcomes of esophageal cancer. PET Clin. 2015;10(2):197–205.
2. Mamede M, El Fakhri G, Abreu-e-Lima P, et al. Preoperative estimation of esophageal tumor metabolic length in FDG-PET images with surgical pathology confirmation. Ann Nucl Med. 2007;21:553–62. 35.
3. Zhong X, Yu J, Zhang B, et al. Using 18F-fluorodeoxyglucose positron emission tomography to estimate the length of gross tumor in patients with squamous cell carcinoma of the esophagus. Int J Radiat Oncol Biol Phys. 2009;73:136–41.
4. Puli SR, Reddy JB, Bechtold ML, Antillon D, Ibdah JA, Antillon MR. Staging accuracy of esophageal cancer by endoscopic ultrasound: a meta-analysis and systematic review. World J Gastroenterol. 2008;14:1479–90.
5. Roedl JB, Blake MA, Holalkere NS, Mueller PR, Colen RR, Harisinghani MG. Lymph node staging in esophageal adenocarcinomas with PET-CT based on a visual analysis and based on metabolic parameters. Abdom Imaging. 2009;34:610–7.
6. Kato H, Kuwano H, Nakajima M, et al. Usefulness of positron emission tomography for assessing the response of neoadjuvant chemoradiotherapy in patients with esophageal cancer. Am J Surg. 2002;184:279–83.
7. Dittrick GW, Weber JM, Shridhar R, et al. Pathologic nonresponders after neoadjuvant chemoradiation for esophageal cancer demonstrate no survival benefit compared with patients treated with primary esophagectomy. Ann Surg Oncol. 2012;19:1678–84. 89.
8. Hsu PK, Chien LI, Huang CS, et al. Comparison of survival among neoadjuvant chemoradiation responders, non-responders and patients receiving primary resection for locally advanced oesophageal squamous cell carcinoma: does neoadjuvant chemoradiation benefit all? Interact Cardiovasc Thorac Surg. 2013;17:460–6.
9. Flamen P, Lerut A, Van Cutsem E, et al. The utility of positron emission tomography for the diagnosis and staging of recurrent esophageal cancer. J Thorac Cardiovasc Surg. 2000;120:1085–92.
10. Cerfolio RJ, Bryant AS, Ohja B, et al. The accuracy of endoscopic ultrasonography with fine-needle aspiration, integrated positron emission tomography with computed tomography, and computed tomography in restaging patients with esophageal cancer after neoadjuvant chemoradiotherapy. J Thorac Cardiovasc Surg. 2005;129:1232–41.
11. Bruzzi JF, Swisher SG, Truong MT, et al. Detection of interval distant metastases: clinical utility of integrated CT-PET imaging in patients with esophageal carcinoma after neoadjuvant therapy. Cancer. 2007;109:125–34.
12. Muijs CT, Beukema JC, Pruim J, et al. A systematic review on the role of FDG-PET/CT in tumour delineation and radiotherapy planning in patients with esophageal cancer. Radiother Oncol. 2010;97:165–71.
13. Shi W, Wang W, Wang J, et al. Meta-analysis of 18FDG PET-CT for nodal staging in patients with esophageal cancer. Surg Oncol. 2013;22:112–6.
14. Yang GY, Wagner TD, Jobe BA, Thomas CR. The role of positron emission tomography in esophageal cancer. Gastrointest Cancer Res. 2008;2(1):3–9.
15. Meyers BF, Downey RJ, Decker PA, American College of Surgeons Oncology Group Z0060, et al. The utility of positron emission tomography in staging of potentially operable carcinoma of the thoracic esophagus: results of the American College of Surgeons Oncology Group Z0060 trial. J Thorac Cardiovasc Surg. 2007;133:738–45.
16. Barber TW, Duong CP, Leong T, et al. 18F-FDG PET/CT has a high impact on patient management and provides powerful prognostic stratification in the primary staging of esophageal cancer: a prospective study with mature survival data. J Nucl Med. 2012;53:864–71.
17. Weber WA, Ott K. Imaging of esophageal and gastric cancer. Semin Oncol. 2004;31:530–41.

18. Walker AJ, Spier BJ, Perlman SB, et al. Integrated PET/CT fusion imaging and endoscopic ultrasound in the pre-operative staging and evaluation of esophageal cancer. Mol Imaging Biol. 2011;13:166–71.
19. Ajani JA, Barthel JS, Bentrem DJ, et al. Esophageal and esophagogastric junction cancers clinical practice guidelines in oncology. J Natl Compr Cancer Netw. 2011;9:830–87.
20. Brigid GA, Flanagan FL, Dehdashti F. Whole-body positron emission tomography: normal variations, pitfalls, and technical considerations. AJR. 1997;169:1675–80.
21. Bruzzi JF, Munden RF, et al. PET/CT of esophageal cancer: its role in clinical management. Radiographics. 2007;27(6):1635–52.
22. Corrigan AJ, Schleyer PJ, et al. Pitfalls and artifacts in the use of PET/CT in oncology imaging. Semin Nucl Med. 2015;45(6):481–99.
23. Sharma R, Mapelli P, Hanna GB, et al. Evaluation of 18F-fluorothymidine positron emission tomography ([18F]FLT-PET/CT) methodology in assessing early response to chemotherapy in patients with gastro-oesophageal cancer. EJNMMI Res. 2016;6(1):81.
24. Vrieze O, Haustermans K, DeWever W, Lerut T, Van Cutsem E, Ectors N, et al. Is there a role for FGD-PET in radiotherapy planning in esophageal carcinoma? Radiother Oncol. 2004;73:269–75.

Gastric Cancer

1. What is the International Gastric Cancer Association classification of gastric cancer at the gastric cardia and gastroesophageal junction ?

   (a) Type I represents a tumor at distal esophagus
   (b) Type II represents a tumor at cardia
   (c) Type III represents a tumor distal to cardia [1]

2. What are the four major histological patterns of gastric cancers recognized by the 2010 World Health Organization classification?

   (a) Tubular (tubular adenocarcinoma is the most common histological type of early gastric carcinoma)
   (b) Papillary
   (c) Mucinous
   (d) Poorly cohesive (including signet ring cell carcinoma)
   (e) Uncommon histologic variants such as adenosquamous carcinoma, squamous carcinoma, hepatoid adenocarcinoma, carcinoma with lymphoid stroma, choriocarcinoma, parietal cell carcinoma, malignant rhabdoid tumor, mucoepidermoid carcinoma, paneth cell carcinoma, undifferentiated carcinoma, mixed adenoneuroendocrine carcinoma, endodermal sinus tumor, embryonal carcinoma, pure gastric yolk sac tumor, and oncocytic adenocarcinoma [2]

3. What are the common indications of ^{18}F-fluorodeoxyglucose (18F-FDG) positron emission tomography (PET)-computed tomography (CT) in gastric cancer?

   The common indications of 18F-FDG PET-CT in gastric cancer are as follows:

   (a) Initial staging—particularly in the detection of distant metastases
   (b) Treatment response assessment
   (c) Detection of recurrent disease/restaging [3–5]

© The Author(s), under exclusive license to Springer Nature Switzerland AG 2026
S. Raja et al., *Question and Answers in PET/CT*,
https://doi.org/10.1007/978-3-032-00821-3_21

4. What is the role of 18F-FDG PET in diagnosis of gastric cancer?

    FDG-PET/CT has a low detection rate (approximately only 55%) for the diagnosis of primary gastric cancer, especially in the early stage, as well as signet-ring cell and mucinous adenocarcinomas, which are typically less metabolically active. Moreover, variable and occasionally intense physiological uptake can mask FDG uptake by the primary tumor [3–5].

5. What is the role of 18F-FDG PET in staging gastric cancer?

    FDG-PET/CT has a limited role in evaluating the T stage. Even though it is more specific for detecting loco-regional lymph nodes, the sensitivity is lower. However, it is more useful in the detection of distant metastases [3–5].

6. What is the role of 18F-FDG PET in re-staging gastric cancer?

    FDG-PET/CT is useful in detecting recurrent disease following a surgical resection procedure, with a recent meta-analysis showing a pooled sensitivity and specificity of 85% and 78%, respectively [6].

7. What is the role of 18F-FDG PET-CT in the assessment of treatment response in gastric cancer?

    18F-FDG PET-CT seems to be useful in identifying responders from non-responders for neoadjuvant chemotherapy in gastric cancer patients with an accuracy of approximately 85% and provides prognostic information as responders have better survival. However, further validation is required in this clinical setting [7].

8. What is the role of 18F-FDG PET-CT in T staging?

    FDG-PET/CT has a limited role in T staging of gastric cancer, particularly at an early stage. It provides very limited information about the involved layer of the gastric wall. The five layers consist of mucosa, submucosa, muscularis, subserosa, and serosa [5, 8].

9. What is the role of 18F-FDG PET-CT in N staging?

    Although FDG-PET/CT is more specific for the detection of loco-regional lymph nodes than CT scanning, it is less sensitive, mainly due to its inability to detect small metastatic lymph nodes, as well as interference by strong photon scatter from an avidly hypermetabolic primary mass. The quoted sensitivity values are typically less than 50% [9]. However, it performs better than CT in detecting distant lymph nodal metastases [8, 10].

10. What is the role of 18F-FDG PET-CT in M staging?

    18F-FDG PET-CT is useful in detecting distant metastases with a pooled sensitivity of around 80% and more than 95% specificity. However, the sensitivity of 18F-FDG PET-CT in detecting peritoneal metastases is very low (only around 30% for all imaging modalities such as EUS, CT, and PET/CT) compared to laparoscopy) [10, 11].

11. What are the common pitfalls of 18F-FDG PET-CT in gastric cancer?

Variable and occasionally intense physiological uptake in the stomach and inflammatory uptake due to gastritis can mask FDG uptake by the primary tumor. Some cancer subtypes like signet ring cell/mucinous adenocarcinomas may be less FDG avid. Due to its limited spatial resolution, FDG PET/CT is not very useful in T staging or detecting loco-regional lymph nodal/ peritoneal metastases [3, 5, 8].

12. What are the common false-positive 18F-FDG PET-CT findings in gastric cancer?

The common false-positive 18F-FDG PET-CT findings include variable physiological FDG uptake in the stomach (which could be overcome by acquiring PET/CT after distending the stomach), infection/ inflammatory conditions such as gastritis, treatment-related changes such as hematoma and post-radiotherapy (RT) inflammation, and so on. In addition, various artifacts such as misregistration artifacts, partial volume effect, attenuation correction artifacts, and truncation artifacts can result in false positives [8, 12, 13].

13. What are the common false-negative 18F-FDG PET-CT findings in gastric cancer?

The common false-negative 18F-FDG PET-CT findings in gastric cancer are

(a) Certain histological sub types are non/less hypermetabolic, such as signet ring cell/ mucinous adenocarcinoma
(b) Small-sized lesions/ lymph nodes (smaller than the resolution of PET scanner), particularly peritoneal and locoregional lymph nodal metastases
(c) Post-chemotherapy status
(d) Artifacts such as misregistration artifacts and so on [8, 12]

14. What are the non-FDG tracers in imaging gastric cancer?

(a) 18F-fluorothymidine (FLT)
(b) 18F-flouromisonidazole
(c) 11C-acetate [14–16]

15. What is the role of 18F-FDG PET-CT in the management of gastric cancer?

18F-FDG PET-CT detects occult distant metastases in around 10% of patients with locally advanced gastric cancer and avoids futile surgeries. In other cases, 18F-FDG PET-CT can detect recurrent disease earlier than CT and guide early treatment [6, 17].

16. What is the role of 18F-FDG PET-CT in RT planning of gastric cancer?

Even though a few studies show that FDG PET-CT may change the gross tumor volume delineation in RT planning of gastric cancer, only limited data is available regarding this, and prospective studies are needed to assess the real impact of the application of PET-CT in RT planning and further clinical outcomes [18].

17. What are the limitations of 18F-FDG PET-CT in RT planning?

Though some gastric tumor subtypes (signet ring cell/mucinous adenocarcinomas) are less FDG avid, 18F-FDG PET-CT may underestimate the disease extent. Several methods (percentage of maximum SUV, fixed SUV cut-off of 2.5, confidence-connected region-growing method, etc.) are being used for tumor volume segmentation. However, the optimal method for tumor volume segmentation is yet to be standardized [18, 19].

18. What is the cost-effectiveness of 18F-FDG PET-CT gastric cancer?

Smyth *et al.* have shown that the addition of FDG-PET/CT to the standard staging evaluation of patients with locally advanced gastric cancer results in an estimated cost savings of ~US $13,000 per patient, as it detects occult metastases in up to 10% of patients and avoids futile surgeries [17].

19. What are the advantages and limitations of 18F-FDG PET-CT in gastric cancer?

Advantages: 18F-FDG PET-CT is useful in detecting distant metastases in patients with locally advanced gastric cancer, as well as detecting suspected recurrence. Early data has demonstrated value in treatment response assessment of gastric cancer and prognostication; however, further studies are required to validate this.

Limitations: A few cancer subtypes like signet ring cell/mucinous adenocarcinomas may be less FDG avid. Due to its limited spatial resolution, FDG PET/CT is not very useful in T staging or detecting loco-regional lymph nodal/ peritoneal metastases [3, 5, 8].

References

1. Siewert JR, Stein HJ. Classification of adenocarcinoma of the oesophagogastric junction. Br J Surg. 1998;85:1457–9.
2. Lauwers GY, Carneiro F, Graham DY. Gastric carcinoma. In: Bowman FT, Carneiro F, Hruban RH, editors. Classification of tumours of the digestive system. Lyon: IARC; 2010.
3. Donswijk ML, Hess S, Mulders T, Lam MG. [18F] Fluorodeoxyglucose PET/computed tomography in gastrointestinal malignancies. PET Clin. 2014;9(4):421–41.
4. Malibari N, Hickeson M, Lisbona R. PET/computed tomography in the diagnosis and staging of gastric cancers. PET Clin. 2015;10(3):311–26.
5. Kitajima K, Nakajo M, Kaida H, et al. Present and future roles of FDG-PET/CT imaging in the management of gastrointestinal cancer: an update. Nagoya J Med Sci. 2017;79(4):527–43.
6. Li P, Liu Q, Wang C, et al. Fluorine-18-fluorodeoxyglucose positron emission tomography to evaluate recurrent gastric cancer after surgical resection: a systematic review and metaanalysis. Ann Nucl Med. 2016;30:179–87.
7. Ott K, Herrmann K, Krause BJ, Lordick F. The value of PET imaging in patients with localized gastroesophageal cancer. Gastrointest Cancer Res. 2008;2:287–94.
8. Gauthé M, Richard-Molard M, Cacheux W, et al. Role of fluorine 18 fluorodeoxyglucose positron emission tomography/computed tomography in gastrointestinal cancers. Dig Liver Dis. 2015;47(6):443–54.
9. Bosch KD, Chicklore S, Cook GJ, et al. Staging FDG PET-CT changes management in patients with gastric adenocarcinoma who are eligible for radical treatment. Eur J Nucl Med Mol Imaging. 2020;47:759–67.

10. Kawanaka Y, Kitajima K, Fukushima K, et al. Added value of pretreatment (18)F-FDG PET/CT for staging of advanced gastric cancer: comparison with contrast-enhanced MDCT. Eur J Radiol. 2016;85(5):989–95.
11. Wang Z, Chen JQ. Imaging in assessing hepatic and peritoneal metastases of gastric cancer: a systematic review. BMC Gastroenterol. 2011;11:19.
12. Corrigan AJ, Schleyer PJ, Cook GJ. Pitfalls and artifacts in the use of PET/CT in oncology imaging. Semin Nucl Med. 2015;45(6):481–99.
13. Eray İC, Rencüzoğulları A, Yalav O, et al. Primary gastric tuberculosis mimicking gastric cancer. Ulus Cerrahi Derg. 2015;31(3):177–9.
14. Nakajo M, Kajiya Y, Tani A, Jinguji M, Nakajo M, Yoshiura T. FLT-PET/CT diagnosis of primary and metastatic nodal lesions of gastric cancer: comparison with FDG-PET/CT. Abdom Radiol (NY). 2016;41(10):1891–8.
15. Staniuk T, Małkowski B, Śrutek E, Szlęzak P, Zegarski W. Comparison of FLT-PET/CT and CECT in gastric cancer diagnosis. Abdom Radiol (NY). 2016;41(7):1349–56.
16. Vardhanabhuti V, Lo AW, Lee EY, Law SY. Dual-tracer PET/CT using 18F-FDG and 11C-acetate in gastric adenocarcinoma with liver metastasis. Clin Nucl Med. 2016;41(11):864–5.
17. Smyth E, Schöder H, Strong VE, et al. A prospective evaluation of the utility of 2-deoxy-2-[(18) F]fluoro-D-glucose positron emission tomography and computed tomography in staging locally advanced gastric cancer. Cancer. 2012;118(22):5481–8.
18. Dębiec K, Wydmański J, Gorczewska I, et al. 18-Fluorodeoxy-glucose positron emission tomography- computed tomography (18-FDG-PET/CT) for gross tumor volume (GTV) delineation in gastric cancer radiotherapy. Asian Pac J Cancer Prev. 2017;18(11):2989–98.
19. Muijs CT, Beukema JC, Pruim J, et al. A systematic review on the role of FDG-PET/CT in tumour delineation and radiotherapy planning in patients with esophageal cancer. Radiother Oncol. 2010;97:165–71.

Prostate Cancer

22

1. What are the common tracers used in prostate imaging?
    The common tracers used in imaging of prostate cancer are as follows:

    (a) Tracer's imaging cell metabolism

        1. Glucose metabolism—18F-fluorodeoxyglucose (FDG)
        2. Cell membrane synthesis—11C-choline/18F-fluorocholine
        3. Fatty acid synthesis—11C-acetate/18F-fluoroacetate
        4. Amino acid metabolism/ transport—18F-anti-1-amino-3-[18F]-fluoro-cyclobutane-1-carboxylic acid (FACBC) (fluciclovine), 11C-methionine, 11C-5-hydroxytryptophan

    (b) Proliferation markers

        1. 18F-fluorothymidine/18F-fluoro-methyl-arabinofuranosyluracil

    (c) Receptor imaging

        1. Androgen Receptor imaging—18F-16β-fluoro-5α-dihydrotestosterone
        2. Gastrin-releasing peptide receptor imaging—68Ga-RM2

    (d) Prostate-specific membrane antigen (PSMA) imaging

        1. Antibody: 111 In-7E11; capromab pendetide [ProstaScint]
        2. Antibody: 99mTc/ 111 In/ 64 Cu/89Zr-J591
        3. Ligand: 68Ga-labeled PSMA ligand or 18F-lableled PSMA ligand

    (e) Imaging of the bone matrix

        1. 99mTc-methylene diphosphonate
        2. 18F-sodium fluoride [1–3]

    (f) Fibroblast-activation-protein (FAP)

        1. 68Ga-labeled—FAP inhibitor (FAPI)

© The Author(s), under exclusive license to Springer Nature
Switzerland AG 2026
S. Raja et al., *Question and Answers in PET/CT*,
https://doi.org/10.1007/978-3-032-00821-3_22

2. What are the common indications of 18F-FDG positron emission tomography (PET)-computed tomography (CT) in prostate cancer?

Because of low FDG avidity, 18F-FDG PET-CT is not used in routine assessment of prostate cancer. However, it gives good prognostic information, particularly in patients with castration-resistant prostate cancer (CRPC). Whenever other tracers for prostate imaging are not available, 18F-FDG PET-CT may have a role in staging aggressive prostate cancer and the detection of recurrent disease in a subgroup of patients with biochemical failure and negative conventional imaging [1, 4].

3. What are the sensitivity and specificity of 18F-FDG PET-CT in diagnosing prostate cancers?

The sensitivity and specificity of 18F-FDG PET-CT in diagnosing prostate cancers are around 50% and 75%, respectively [5].

4. What are common pitfalls of 18F-FDG PET-CT in staging prostate cancer?

FDG uptake in prostate cancer and its metastases are usually less due to the low rate of glycolysis. Overlap of FDG uptake exists in normal prostate, benign prostate hyperplasia (BPH), and prostate cancer tissues. In addition, there is interference by high urinary tracer activity in the bladder while assessing the T stage of the disease and detecting locoregional recurrence [4].

5. What are the common false-positive 18F-FDG PET-CT findings in prostate cancer?

The common false-positive 18F-FDG PET-CT findings in prostate cancer are as follows:

(a) FDG uptake in normal prostate, BPH, and prostatitis may mimic tumoral uptake.
(b) Physiological FDG uptake in the intestine or urinary tracer activity in the bladder may result in false positivity.
(c) Treatment-related changes like post-radiotherapy/surgery inflammatory changes, and so on.
(d) In addition, various artifacts such as misregistration artifact, partial volume effect, attenuation correction artifact, and truncation artifact can result in false positives [4, 6].

6. What are the common false-negative 18F-FDG PET-CT findings in prostate cancer?

The common false-negative 18F-FDG PET-CT findings in prostate cancer are as follows:

1. Most prostate cancer patients show low FDG avidity, resulting in false-negative findings due to its indolent nature
2. Small-sized lesions/lymph nodes (smaller than the resolution of the PET scanner)
3. Post-chemotherapy status/androgen deprivation therapy (ADT) (could decrease the FDG uptake by tumor cells)
4. Artifacts like misregistration artifacts and so on [4, 6]

7. What is the cost-effectiveness of 18F-FDG PET-CT in prostate cancer?

Because of its low sensitivity, routine use of 18F-FDG PET-CT in the assessment of prostate cancer is not cost-effective.

8. What are the advantages and limitations of 18F-FDG PET-CT in prostate cancer?

Advantages:

(a) 18F-FDG PET-CT may be useful in staging and detection of recurrent disease in a subset of patients with aggressive prostate cancer where other radiotracers are not available.
(b) Good prognostic information.

Limitations:

(a) FDG uptake in prostate cancer and its metastases are usually less due to a low rate of glycolysis.
(b) Overlap of FDG uptake in normal prostate, BPH, and prostate cancer tissues.
(c) Interference by high tracer activity in the urinary bladder while assessing locoregional disease [1–3].

9. What are common indications of 11C/18F-Choline PET-CT in staging prostate cancer?

Choline PET-CT is useful in the detection of locoregional lymph nodal or distant metastatic disease in patients with biochemical recurrence. It may also have a role in detecting distant metastases during initial staging and treatment response assessment in CRPC. It is not useful in the detection of primary prostate cancer or lymph nodal metastases during initial staging [1, 2].

10. What are the sensitivity and specificity of 18F-Choline PET-CT in detecting prostate cancers?

Even though choline PET-CT is relatively more specific (usually around 85%) in the detection of prostate cancer, its sensitivity is low (only around 55–65%) [7, 8].

11. What are the sensitivity and specificity of Choline PET-CT in the assessment of nodal disease in prostate cancer?

Even though choline PET-CT is highly specific (usually >95%) in the assessment of nodal disease in prostate cancer, its sensitivity is low (around 50%) [9].

12. What are the sensitivity and specificity of Choline PET-CT in the assessment of bone metastasis?

The pooled sensitivity and specificity of Choline PET-CT in detecting prostate cancer bone metastasis are 84% and 93%, respectively [10].

13. What is the role of Choline PET-CT in re-staging prostate cancer?

Choline PET-CT is useful in detecting recurrent disease, particularly in patients who demonstrate significantly elevated prostate membrane antigen (PSA) levels or fast PSA kinetics with pooled sensitivity and specificity for detecting all sites of recurrent disease being 86% and 93%, respectively. The pooled sensitivity and specificity for detecting prostatic fossa recurrence are 75% and 82%, and for lymph node recurrence, they are 100% and 82%, respectively. However, its sensitivity is very low (only around 20%) in patients with PSA values <1 ng/mL [11].

14. What is the role of Choline PET-CT in the assessment of treatment response in prostate cancer?

Choline PET-CT may help assess therapy response, especially in CRPC patients whose PSA value is not predictive of disease burden [2, 12].

15. What are the common pitfalls of Choline PET-CT in the evaluation of prostate cancer?

The common pitfalls of Choline PET-CT in the evaluation of prostate cancer are as follows:

(a) Physiological Choline uptake is in various organs such as salivary glands, liver, kidney parenchyma, and pancreas, as well as faint uptake in the spleen, bone marrow, and muscles. This results in relatively high background activity and low target-to-background activity ratios [13].
(b) Relatively high image noise levels [13].
(c) Choline uptake is not specific to prostate cancer and may also be observed in inflammatory processes, BPH, benign tumors, and other synchronous malignant disease.
(d) 18F-Fluorocholine may be excreted in urine and interfere with the assessment of local disease.
(e) ADT may reduce choline uptake in androgen-sensitive prostate cancer patients [1, 6, 14, 15].

16. What are the common false-positive Choline PET-CT findings in prostate cancer?

The common false-positive Choline PET-CT findings in prostate cancer are as follows:

(a) Physiological Choline uptake is in various organs such as salivary glands, liver, kidney parenchyma, and pancreas, as well as faint uptake in the spleen, bone marrow, and muscles, urinary tracer activity in case of 18F-fluorocholine PET.
(b) Choline uptake may be observed in inflammatory processes, BPH, benign tumors, and other synchronous malignant disease.
(c) Treatment-related changes such as post-radiotherapy/surgery inflammatory changes, and so on.
(d) In addition, various artifacts such as misregistration artifact, partial volume effect, attenuation correction artifact, and truncation artifact can result in false positives [6].

17. What are the common false-negative Choline PET findings in prostate cancer?

The common false-negative Choline PET findings in prostate cancer are as follows:

(a) Choline PET may be falsely negative in a significant number of patients with prostate cancer, mainly if serum PSA levels are low or in patients with slow PSA kinetics.

(b) Small-sized lesions/lymph nodes (smaller than the resolution of the PET scanner)

(c) Post-chemotherapy status/ADT (could decrease the choline uptake by tumor cells)

(d) Artifacts such as misregistration artifacts and so on [6, 14, 15]

18. What is the cost-effectiveness of Choline PET-CT in prostate cancer?

Routine use of Choline PET-CT in the detection and staging of prostate cancer is not cost-effective [16, 17].

19. What is the mechanism of PSMA imaging in prostate cancer?

PSMA is a type II transmembrane glycoprotein encoded by the folate hydrolase 1 gene, also called the glutamate carboxypeptidase II gene. This is expressed in normal prostate tissue and is overexpressed in prostate cancer. PSMA expression appears to be progressively increased in higher-grade prostate cancers, under androgen deprivation, and in hormone-refractory and metastatic disease.

Small molecules that bind to the extracellular active center of PSMA are labeled with Gallium-68. Compared with anti-PSMA antibodies (e.g., 111-In Capromab/ 89Zr-J591), 68Ga-PSMA ligands (68Ga-PSMA-11, 68Ga-PSMA-617, and 68Ga-PSMA-I&T) have the advantages of higher binding affinity, internalization, and rapid plasma clearance [18]. The majority of published studies used 68Ga-labeling for PSMA PET imaging, but some used 18F-labeling. At present, there is no conclusive data on the comparison of such tracers. 68Ga-labeled or 18F-labeled radiotracers for PSMA PET/CT imaging provide a good contrast-to-noise ratio, thereby improving the detectability of lesions [18].

Due to magnetic resonance imaging (MRI)'s superior soft tissue contrast resolution property, 68Ga-PSMA PET/MRI enables the practical potential of multimodal, combined metabolic-receptor, anatomical, and functional imaging.

20. What is the normal physiological distribution of 68Ga-PSMA?

Physiologic high-intensity activity is seen in the lacrimal, parotid, and submandibular glands and the small intestine, primarily in the duodenum.

Moderate-intensity uptake is seen in the liver and spleen.

Low PSMA uptake is also seen in the parasympathetic ganglia, most commonly in the celiac and stellate ganglia and the presacral ganglia.

The highest intensity uptake is seen in the kidneys, ureters, and bladder, as it is renally excreted. 68Ga-PSMA is also minimally excreted in saliva, which may result in oropharyngeal, laryngeal, or esophagal uptake [19].

21. What are the common indications of 68Ga-PSMA PET-CT in prostate cancer?

PSMA PET-CT is rapidly emerging as a potential new reference standard for prostate cancer imaging, with extraordinary tumor-to-background contrast.

It has been shown to be very useful in the primary staging of high-risk prostate cancer and localization of disease in patients with biochemical recurrence, even if the PSA values are very low. 68Ga-PSMA PET-CT may play a role in the response assessment of prostate cancer following systemic therapy/ radioligand therapy targeting PSMA.

It may also help guide focal therapy (such as ablation by radiofrequency, laser, cryotherapy, electroporation, etc.) as well as biopsy to establish cancer diagnosis, particularly after a previous negative biopsy but with high suspicion for prostate cancer.

68Ga-PSMA PET-CT is also helpful in selecting patients for Lu-177 PSMA therapy [3, 19].

22. What is the role of ^{68}Ga-PSMA PET in staging prostate cancer?

68Ga-PSMA PET-CT appears to be more accurate in the staging of prostate cancer, particularly in high-risk patients (according to D'Amico risk classification, if at least one of the following three features exists: PSA level greater than 20, Gleason score greater than 8, or clinical stage of T2c or T3a). However, its role in staging low- to intermediate-risk prostate cancers seems to be of limited value [19–21].

PSMA PET-MRI-guided biopsy has been described, but studies are needed to elucidate the advantages of diagnostic efficiency and costs compared to the more established MRI-TRUS fusion biopsy [22].

23. What is the role of 68Ga-PSMA PET-CT in re-staging prostate cancer?

68Ga-PSMA PET-CT is useful and more accurate than Choline PET-CT, considered the best PET tracer until recently, in identifying disease sites in patients with biochemical recurrence, even if PSA levels are low (<1 ng/mL). It detects recurrent disease in a significant number (>40%) of choline PET-negative patients [19, 23–25].

24. What is the role of 68Ga-PSMA PET-CT in the assessment of treatment response in prostate cancer?

Early studies showed that 68Ga-PSMA PET-CT may play a role in the response assessment of prostate cancer following systemic therapy/radioligand therapy targeting PSMA. However, more data is needed in this clinical setting. Readers should be aware of the "Flare" phenomenon with PSMA PET following ADT. ADT has been reported to result in transient amplified PSMA expression [19, 26]. The increased PSMA ligand uptake can co-exist with successful treatment and induced cell death-related decrease in tumor size [27]. It is thought that long-term ADT decreases PSMA-ligand uptake as tumor volume changes.

25. What are the sensitivity and specificity of 68Ga-PSMA PET in detecting pros-
    tate cancer?

    A recent meta-analysis showed pooled sensitivity and specificity for prostate
    cancer detection to be 70% and 84% [28]. Another systematic review found
    patient-based primary tumor pooled sensitivity to be 94.9% and detection rate
    to be 80.9% at restaging [22].

26. What are the sensitivity and specificity of 68Ga-PSMA PET-CT in the assess-
    ment of nodal disease in prostate cancer?

    A recent meta-analysis showed pooled sensitivity and specificity of 61% and
    97% in the assessment of nodal disease in prostate cancer [28].

27. What are the sensitivity and specificity of 68Ga-PSMA PET-CT in the assess-
    ment of metastasis in prostate cancer?

    The most common sites of hematogenous metastases are bone, lung, liver,
    pleura, and adrenal glands. Initial studies showed superior sensitivity and speci-
    ficity (>95%) of 68Ga-PSMA PET-CT for detecting osseous metastases in
    patients with prostate cancer compared to conventional imaging methods such
    as bone scintigraphy with single-photon emission computed tomography
    (SPECT)/CT or Choline PET-CT. However, data is limited, and further prop-
    erly designed studies are needed to clarify the diagnostic performance and
    superiority over existing methods and their clinical implications [29–32].

28. What are the common pitfalls of 68Ga-PSMA PET-CT in staging of
    prostate cancer?

    Despite the term "prostate specific," PSMA is functionally an enzyme
    (folate hydrolase) expressed in various normal tissues, tissue neovasculature,
    inflammation/infection, and other benign and malignant tumor types, which
    may result in false positivity.

    Urinary excretion of tracer can interfere with the evaluation of prostate/
    prostatic bed lesions or pelvic and retroperitoneal lymph nodes.

    Neuroendocrine differentiation and dedifferentiation of prostate cancer in
    metastases can result in low PSMA expression [19, 33]. This is seen in advanced
    stages and following lasting ADT. In addition, tumor heterogeneity can result in
    variable PSMA expression between metastases [33]. FAPI PET has been pro-
    posed to improve diagnostic accuracy in this cohort [34].

29. What are the common false-positive 68Ga-PSMA PET-CT findings in
    prostate cancer?

    The common false-positive 68Ga-PSMA PET–CT findings in prostate
    cancer are as follows:

    (a) Physiological PSMA uptake in various organs as mentioned above (e.g.,
        coeliac ganglionic uptake may be mistaken as lymph nodal metastases) and
        excreted urinary tracer activity may lead to false positivity.
    (b) PSMA uptake may be observed in various benign conditions such as infec-
        tion, inflammation, osteoarthritis, degenerative changes, fibrous dysplasia,
        Paget's disease, gynecomastia, tuberculosis, fracture, hemangioma, menin-
        gioma, and so on.

(c) High-intensity PSMA uptake is seen in soft tissue tumors such as thymomas and adenomas and synchronous malignancies, including renal cell carcinoma, salivary gland ductal carcinoma, pulmonary adenocarcinoma, glioblastoma multiforme, breast cancer, hepatocellular carcinoma, lymphoma, squamous cell carcinoma, and well-differentiated thyroid cancer.
(d) Treatment-related changes such as flare phenomenon following ADT, post-radiotherapy/surgery inflammatory changes, and so on.
(e) In addition, various artifacts such as misregistration artifact, partial volume effect, attenuation correction artifact, and truncation artifact can result in false positives [1, 6, 19, 35, 36].

30. What are the common false-negative 68Ga-PSMA PET-CT findings in prostate cancer?

The common false-negative 68Ga-PSMA PET-CT findings in prostate cancer are as follows:

(a) PSMA PET CT may be falsely negative in a small number (approximately 5–10%) of prostate cancer patients, such as poorly differentiated type with neuroendocrine differentiation.
(b) Even though it detects many subcentimetric lesions, sensitivity falls when lesion/lymph node size falls below 1 cm. Notably, 91% of lymph node metastases <5 mm in diameter, and all metastatic lymph nodes <2 mm were undetectable by PSMA PET-CT [37].
(c) Halo effect around organs (e.g., ureters and bladder) demonstrating intense tracer uptake may obscure/mask adjacent lesions.
(d) Artifacts such as misregistration artifacts and metal artifacts from prostatic radiotherapy fiducials, and so on [6, 19].
(e) False negatives are more common in patients with lower serum PSA values or slower PSA kinetics. Intraductal prostate cancer has been shown to have a lower PSA expression by 30% [38].

31. What is the cost-effectiveness of 68Ga-PSMA PET-CT in prostate cancer?

No significant published data is available regarding the cost-effectiveness of PSMA PET-CT in prostate cancer in different settings. Cost saving has been demonstrated in preliminary data concerning initial prostate cancer staging, treatment planning, and biochemical recurrence staging [39–42].

32. What are the advantages and limitations of 68Ga-PSMA PET-CT in prostate cancer?

Advantages: Due to its extraordinary tumor-to-background ratio and higher sensitivity and specificity, 68Ga-PSMA PET-CT is emerging as a new reference standard for prostate cancer imaging, particularly for staging of high-grade prostate cancer and detecting disease sites in patients with biochemical recurrence.

Limitations: Despite prostate-specific terminology, PSMA is expressed in a range of normal tissues and other benign and malignant processes (Knowledge of the physiologic distribution and benign uptake causes will minimize false-positive findings). Data on the implications of PSMA PET/CT to improve patient-related outcomes, particularly in early biochemical recurrence and targeted treatment of oligo-metastatic disease, are limited. PSMA uptake may be absent in poorly differentiated prostate cancer with neuroendocrine differentiation [1, 19].

33. What is the role of 18F-fluoride PET-CT in the assessment of skeletal metastases?

    18F-fluoride PET-CT is more accurate than a conventional bone scan (the most commonly performed investigation in routine clinical practice) for detecting osseous metastases in prostate cancer with a pooled sensitivity and specificity of approximately 89% and 90%, respectively [43, 44].

34. What are the advantages and limitations of 18F-fluoride PET-CT in prostate cancer?

    Advantages: 18F-fluoride PET-CT is more accurate than a conventional bone scan for detecting osseous metastases in prostate cancer. Compared to bone scan, it has some advantages such as less plasma protein binding with resultant higher bone uptake and faster serum clearance as well as shorter uptake time (30–45 min instead of 2–3 h), greater spatial resolution (4–5 mm instead of 10–15 mm), higher sensitivity, and better image quality with higher target-to-background ratio.

    Limitations: Even though 18F-fluoride PET-CT is highly sensitive, its specificity is limited, as it is only a surrogate marker of bone metastases (increased uptake is seen in various benign conditions with increased perfusion or bone turnover rate). Thus, higher uptake might be seen in cases of tumor regression with ongoing bone formation, the so-called "flare" phenomenon, particularly following hormonal therapy. Since it is a pure bone-seeking agent, 18F-fluoride PET-CT is not useful in detecting visceral metastases. More prospective studies are needed comparing 18F-fluoride and other new tracers like choline/PSMA and their overall implications on patient management [1, 43, 44].

References

1. Wibmer AG, Burger IA, Sala E, Hricak H, Weber WA, Vargas HA. Molecular imaging of prostate cancer. Radiographics. 2016;36(1):142–59.
2. Schuster DM, Nanni C, Fanti S. PET tracers beyond FDG in prostate cancer. Semin Nucl Med. 2016;46(6):507–21.
3. Bouchelouche K, Turkbey B, Choyke PL. PSMA PET and radionuclide therapy in prostate cancer. Semin Nucl Med. 2016;46(6):522–35.
4. Jadvar H. Is there use for FDG-PET in prostate cancer? Semin Nucl Med. 2016;46(6):502–6.
5. Minamimoto R, Uemura H, Sano F, et al. The potential of FDG PET/CT for detecting prostate cancer in patients with an elevated serum PSA level. Ann Nucl Med. 2011;25:21–7.
6. Corrigan AJ, Schleyer PJ, Cook GJ. Pitfalls and artifacts in the use of PET/CT in oncology imaging. Semin Nucl Med. 2015;45(6):481–99.
7. Testa C, Schiavina R, Lodi R, et al. Prostate cancer: sextant localization with MR imaging. MR spectroscopy, and 11C-choline PET-CT. Radiology. 2007;244(3):797–806.

8. Farsad M, Schiavina R, Castellucci P, et al. Detection and localization of prostate cancer: correlation of 11C-choline PET-CT with histopathologic step-section analysis. J Nucl Med. 2005;46(10):1642–9.
9. Evangelista L, Guttilla A, Zattoni F, Muzzio PC, Zattoni F. Utility of choline positron emission tomography/computed tomography for lymph node involvement identifcation in intermediate- to high-risk prostate cancer: a systematic literature review and meta-analysis. Eur Urol. 2013;63(6):1040–8.
10. Shen G, Deng H, Hu S, et al. Comparison of choline-PET/CT, MRI, SPECT, and bone scintigraphy in the diagnosis of bone metastases in patients with prostate cancer: a meta-analysis. Skeletal Radiol. 2014;43:1503–13.
11. Evangelista L, Zattoni F, Guttilla A, et al. Choline PET or PET/CT and biochemical relapse of prostate cancer: a systematic review and meta-analysis. Clin Nucl Med. 2013;38(5):305–14.
12. Ceci F, Castellucci P, Graziani T, et al. 11 C-Choline PET-CT in castration-resistant prostate cancer patients treated with docetaxel. Eur J Nucl Med Mol Imaging. 2016;43(1):84–91.
13. Michaud L, Touijer KA, Maugein A, et al. 11C-Choline PET/CT in recurrent prostate cancer: retrospective analysis in a large U.S. patient series. J Nucl Med. 2020;61(6):827–33.
14. Fuccio C, Schiavina R, Castellucci P, et al. Androgen deprivation therapy influences the uptake of 11C-choline in patients with recurrent prostate cancer: the preliminary results of a sequential PET-CT study. Eur J Nucl Med Mol Imaging. 2011;38(11):1985–9.
15. Emonds KM, Swinnen JV, Lerut E, Koole M, Mortelmans L, Mottaghy FM. Evaluation of androgen-induced effects on the uptake of [18F]FDG, [11C]choline and [11C]acetate in an androgen-sensitive and androgen-independent prostate cancer xenograft model. EJNMMI Res. 2013;3(1):31.
16. Kjölhede H, Almquist H, Lyttkens K, Bratt O. A population-based study of the clinical utility of 18F–choline PET/CT for primary metastasis staging of high-risk prostate cancer. Eur J Hybrid Imaging. 2017;1:12.
17. Nitsch S, Hakenberg OW, Heuschkel M, et al. Evaluation of prostate cancer with 11C- and 18F-Choline PET/CT: diagnosis and initial staging. J Nucl Med. 2016;57(Suppl 3):38S–42S.
18. EAU Guidelines. Edn. presented at the EAU Annual Congress Milan 2021. ISBN 978-94-92671-13-4.
19. Hofman MS, Hicks RJ, Maurer T, Eiber M. Prostate-specific membrane antigen PET: clinical utility in prostate cancer, normal patterns, pearls, and pitfalls. Radiographics. 2018;38(1):200–17.
20. Maurer T, Gschwend JE, Rauscher I, et al. Diagnostic effcacy of (68)gallium-PSMA positron emission tomography compared to conventional imaging for lymph node staging of 130 consecutive patients with intermediate to high risk prostate cancer. J Urol. 2016;195(5):1436–43.
21. Herlemann A, Wenter V, Kretschmer A, et al. (68)Ga-PSMA positron emission tomography/computed tomography provides accurate staging of lymph node regions prior to lymph node dissection in patients with prostate cancer. Eur Urol. 2016;70(4):553–7.
22. Evangelista L, Zattoni F, Cassarino G, et al. PET/MRI in prostate cancer: a systematic review and meta-analysis. Eur J Nucl Med Mol Imaging. 2021;48:859–73.
23. Perera M, Papa N, Christidis D, et al. Sensitivity, specifcity, and predictors of positive (68) Ga-prostate-specifc membrane antigen positron emission tomography in advanced prostate cancer: a systematic review and meta-analysis. Eur Urol. 2016;70(6):926–37.
24. Afshar-Oromieh A, Zechmann CM, Malcher A, et al. Comparison of PET imaging with a (68)Ga-labeled PSMA ligand and (18)F-choline-based PET/CT for the diagnosis of recurrent prostate cancer. Eur J Nucl Med Mol Imaging. 2014;41(1):11–20.
25. Bluemel C, Krebs M, Polat B, et al. 68Ga-PSMA-PET/CT in patients with biochemical prostate cancer recurrence and negative 18F-Choline-PET/ CT. Clin Nucl Med. 2016;41:515–21.
26. Afshar-Oromieh A, Malcher A, Eder M, et al. Reply to Reske et al: PET imaging with a [68Ga]gallium-labelled PSMA ligand for the diagnosis of prostate cancer: biodistribution in humans and frst evaluation of tumour lesions. Eur J Nucl Med Mol Imaging. 2013;40(6):971–2.
27. Vaz S, Hadaschik B, Gabriel M, et al. Influence of androgen deprivation therapy on PSMA expression and PSMA-ligand PET imaging of prostate cancer patients. Eur J Nucl Med Mol Imaging. 2020;47:9–15. https://doi.org/10.1007/s00259-019-04529-8.

28. von Eyben FE, Picchio M, von Eyben R, Rhee H, Bauman G. 68Ga-labeled prostate-specific membrane antigen ligand positron emission tomography/computed tomography for prostate cancer: a systematic review and meta-analysis. Eur Urol Focus. 2016. pii: S2405-4569.

29. Pyka T, Okamoto S, Dahlbender M, et al. Comparison of bone scintigraphy and 68Ga-PSMA PET for skeletal staging in prostate cancer. Eur J Nucl Med Mol Imaging. 2016;43(12):2114–21.

30. Janssen JC, Meißner S, Woythal N, et al. Comparison of hybrid 68Ga-PSMA-PET/CT and 99mTc-DPD-SPECT/CT for the detection of bone metastases in prostate cancer patients: Additional value of morphologic information from low dose CT. Eur Radiol. 2018;28(2):610–9.

31. Schwenck J, Rempp H, Reischl G, et al. Comparison of 68Ga-labelled PSMA-11 and 11C-choline in the detection of prostate cancer metastases by PET/CT. Eur J Nucl Med Mol Imaging. 2017;44(1):92–101.

32. Zacho HD, Nielsen JB, Haberkorn U, Stenholt L, Petersen LJ. 68 Ga-PSMA PET/CT for the detection of bone metastases in prostate cancer: a systematic review of the published literature. Clin Physiol Funct Imaging. 2017; https://doi.org/10.1111/cpf.12480. [Epub ahead of print].

33. Seifert R, Seitzer K, Herrmann K, et al. Analysis of PSMA expression and outcome in patients with advanced prostate cancer receiving ^{177}Lu-PSMA-617 Radioligand Therapy. Theranostics. 2020;10(17):7812–20. Published 2020 Jun 19. https://doi.org/10.7150/thno.47251.

34. Laudicella R, Spataro A, Crocè L, Giacoppo G, Romano D, Davì V, Lopes M, Librando M, Nicocia A, Rappazzo A, Celesti G, Torre FL, Pagano B, Garraffa G, Bauckneht M, Burger IA, Minutoli F, Baldari S. Preliminary findings of the role of FAPi in prostate cancer theranostics. Diagnostics. 2023;13(6):1175. https://doi.org/10.3390/diagnostics13061175.

35. Sasikumar A, Joy A, Nair BP, Pillai MRA, Madhavan J. False positive uptake in bilateral gynecomastia on 68Ga-PSMA PET/CT scan. Clin Nucl Med. 2017;42(9):e412–4.

36. Sathekge M, Lengana T, Modiselle M, et al. 68Ga-PSMA-HBED-CC PET imaging in breast carcinoma patients. Eur J Nucl Med Mol Imaging. 2017;44(4):689–94.

37. van Leeuwen PJ, Emmett L, Ho B, Delprado W, Ting F, Nguyen Q, Stricker PD. evaluation of 68Gallium-prostate-specific membrane antigen positron emission tomography/computed tomography for preoperative lymph node staging in prostate cancer. BJU Int. 2017;119:209–15. https://doi.org/10.1111/bju.13540.

38. Morgan TM, Welty CJ, Vakar-Lopez F, Lin DW, Wright JL. Ductal adenocarcinoma of the prostate: Increased mortality risk and decreased serum prostate specific antigen. J Urol. 2010;184:2303–7.

39. van der Sar ECA, Keusters WR, van Kalmthout LWM, et al. Cost-effectiveness of the implementation of [^{68}Ga]Ga-PSMA-11 PET/CT at initial prostate cancer staging. Insights Imaging. 2022;13:132. https://doi.org/10.1186/s13244-022-01265-w.

40. Rovera G, Oprea-Lager DE, Ceci F. Health technology assessment for PSMA-PET: striving towards a cost-effective management of prostate cancer. Clin Translat Imaging. 2021;9:409–12. https://doi.org/10.1007/s40336-021-00446-9.

41. Gordon LG, Elliott TM, Joshi A, et al. Exploratory cost-effectiveness analysis of [68]Gallium-PSMA PET/MRI-based imaging in patients with biochemical recurrence of prostate cancer. Clin Exp Metastasis. 2020;37:305–12. https://doi.org/10.1007/s10585-020-10027-1.

42. Wondergem M, van der Zant FM, van der Ploeg T, Knol RJ. A literature review of 18F-fluoride PET/CT and 18F-choline or 11C-choline PET/CT for detection of bone metastases in patients with prostate cancer. Nucl Med Commun. 2013;34(10):935–45.

43. Langsteger W, Rezaee A, Pirich C, Beheshti M. 18F-NaF-PET/CT and 99mTc-MDP Bone Scintigraphy in the Detection of Bone Metastases in Prostate Cancer. Semin Nucl Med. 2016;46(6):491–501.

44. Mei R, Farolfi A, Castellucci P, Nanni C, Zanoni L, Fanti S. PET/CT variants and pitfalls in prostate cancer: what you might see on PET and should never forget. Semin Nucl Med. 2021;51(6):621–32.

Multiple Myeloma

23

1. What is multiple myeloma (MM)?

   MM is a neoplastic disease characterized by the proliferation and accumulation of B-lymphocytes and plasma cells (PCs), which synthesize monoclonal immunoglobulin (M-protein or paraprotein) in the bone marrow (BM) or, more rarely, in extramedullary tissues [1]. MM is a heterogeneous and complex disease and can be stratified into two subgroups based upon the prevalent recurring genomic aberrations identified by fluorescence *in situ* hybridization: (a) hyperdiploid (H) karyotype and (b) non-hyper-diploid karyotype (NH) [1, 2].

2. What are the common features of plasma cell disorders (PCDs)?

   The common feature of all PCDs is the production and secretion of an M-protein. The M-protein is an intact immunoglobulin (IgG, IgA, or rarely IgD or IgM) which can be quantified and specified by serum electrophoresis and immunofixation [1].

3. What are the CRAB criteria in MM?

   Hypercalcemia, renal insufficiency, anemia, and bone lesion (1 osteolytic lesion, 5 mm in size on X-ray, computed tomography (CT) or CT component of positron emission tomography (PET)-CT) [1, 2].

4. What is non-secretory MM?

   In approximately 1–2% of MM patients where no paraprotein is produced is called non-secretory MM [1].

5. What is the definition of smoldering MM (SMM)?

   SMM is defined as clonal PC proliferation with 10–60% of PCs in the BM without organ damage. The risk of SMM progressing to MM is ~10% each year during the first 5 years [3, 4].

© The Author(s), under exclusive license to Springer Nature
Switzerland AG 2026
S. Raja et al., *Question and Answers in PET/CT*,
https://doi.org/10.1007/978-3-032-00821-3_23

6. What are PET radiopharmaceuticals in MM?

   PET radiopharmaceuticals in imaging MM include ^{18}F-fluorodeoxyglucose (18F-FDG), 18F-NaF, 68Ga-Pentixafor, and 11C-Choline [1].

7. What is the role of radiological imaging in myeloma?

   The primary role of imaging in MM is to identify sites of bone disease that necessitate starting treatment [1, 2].

8. What is myeloma-related bone disease?

   Myeloma-related bone disease is defined as the presence of one or more osteolytic bone lesions (≥5 mm) attributable to an underlying clonal PCD [3, 4].

9. What is the current International Myeloma Working Group (IMWG) recommendations for imaging monoclonal gammopathy of unknown significance (MGUS) and for SMM?

   The IMWG recommends WB-LDCT as first-line imaging for suspected MGUS and SMM [1, 2].

10. What are the current IMWG recommendations for imaging MM?

    The IMWG recommends WB-LDCT or 18F-FDG PET-CT imaging for suspected MM. WB-MRI is recommended if there are inconclusive findings on prior whole-body imaging [1, 2].

11. What are the current IMWG recommendations for imaging suspected plasmacytoma?

    The IMWG recommends WB-MRI as the first-line for suspected solitary plasmacytoma (SP) of the bone, while 18F-FDG PET-CT is the first line for suspected extramedullary SP [3, 5, 6].

12. What are the advantages and limitations of Plain radiography?

    Historically, radiographic skeletal surveys have been used for many years to detect the occurrence of osteolytic lesions in patients with MM. In general, a complete skeletal survey is performed in patients suspected of myeloma (frontal and lateral views of the skull, cervical, thoracic, and lumbar spine, a coned-down frontal view of the dens axis, frontal views of the rib cage, humeri, femora, knees, and pelvis) [Healy CF, Durie BGM]. The advantages of plain radiography include the detection of cortical bone lesions, availability, and low cost. The limitations include low sensitivity of radiographs for the detection of osteolytic bone disease, high false-negative rate (30–70%), [1, 7–10], and inability to assess BM-based disease [1].

13. What are the advantages and limitations of CT?

    The IMWG recommends WB-LDCT as the first line for suspected MGUS and SMM and either WB-LDCT or 18F-FDG PET/CT for suspected MM [5]. CT is sensitive in detecting the osteolytic lesions of MM. CT is more sensitive than plain radiography at detecting small lytic lesions [7, 11]. The other advantages of CT include accurately evaluating areas at risk of fracture, identifying bone destruction in cases where MR is negative, detecting the presence and extent of extraosseous lesions and image-guided bone biopsy [12]. The limitations of CT include high radiation exposure and often show persistent bone lesions throughout the disease [12].

14. What are the advantages and limitations of MRI imaging?

Whole-body MRI is the most sensitive imaging modality in detecting diffuse and focal MM in the spine, the extra-axial skeleton, and the ability to visualize large volumes of BM without radiation exposure [13–15]. The limitations of MRI include limited specificity. Focal or diffuse patterns may exist at diagnosis or reflect an alternative pathological or physiological process.

15. What is the field of view of PET-CT in patients with MM?

The CT and PET acquisitions should be conducted from the skull vertex to the toes (or at least to the knees) [1].

16. What is the role of 18FDG PET/CT for initial diagnosis and staging?

18F-FDG PET-CT is useful in detecting osteolytic bone lesions >5 mm, a CRAB criterion [16].

17. What is the role of 18F-FDG PET-CT in MM?

1. Detection of both medullary and extramedullary disease (EMD)
2. Assessment of disease burden of the disease.
3. To evaluate and monitor response to treatment (e.g., distinguish metabolically active and inactive lesions)
4. To determine the prognosis in patients with newly diagnosed and relapsed or refractory MM [1, 2]

18. What are the advantages of 18F-FDG PET-CT in MM?

1. 18F-FDG PET/CT is a powerful tool for evaluating tumor activity and metabolic response to therapy.
2. 18F-FDG PET/CT is recommended for the work-up of newly diagnosed and relapsed or refractory MM.
3. Negative 18F-FDG PET/CT scans after treatment predict better outcomes in patients who achieved complete response after autologous stem-cell transplantation.
4. 18F-FDG PET/CT is useful to distinguish smoldering MM from active MM if a whole-body X-ray is negative and a whole-body MRI is unavailable.
5. 18F-FDG PET/CT is of high value in diagnosing and assessing SP.
6. 18F-FDG PET/CT is useful in assessing the extent of response to treatment and detecting disease recurrence early in MM patients [1, 2].

19. What is the role of 18F-FDG PET/CT in the staging of MM?

18F-FDG PET-CT has higher screening and diagnostic sensitivity and specificity over the skeleton X-ray [17, 18]. 18F-FDG PET/CT enables high sensitivity and reasonable specificity for the detection of both medullary and EMD [1, 2].

20. What are the sensitivity and specificity of 18F-FDG PET-CT in the detection of MM lesions?

    18F-FDG PET-CT has a sensitivity of 90% and specificity of 70–100% in detecting MM lesions [19–21].

21. What are the sensitivity and specificity of 18F-FDG PET/CT in the staging of MM?

    18F-FDG PET/CT represents a modality of choice in the various phases of MM: studies in the literature report a high sensitivity and specificity, ranging from 80% to 100%, in evaluating BM and EMD [22–24]. 18F-FDG is useful to assess the disease's burden and distinguish between metabolically active and inactive lesions [2].

22. What is the role of 18F-FDG PET-CT in disease detection in symptomatic MM?

    In the prospective multicentric Cassio PET study, 18F-FDG PET-CT was normal at diagnosis for 20% of patients, 67% had FLs, 48% had diffuse BM infiltration, and 8% had EMD. The sensitivity of 18F-FDG PET-CT for symptomatic MM is comparable/less than pelvic-spinal MRI (PSMRI) [25–27]. 18F-FDG PET-CT sensitivity was lower than PSMRI for diffuse BM involvement. WBMRI with DWI improves the sensitivity for FL detection, which is higher than 18F-FDG PET/CT, especially in SMM patients at initial diagnosis.

23. What are the IMWG consensus recommendations for the optimal use of 18F-FDG PET/CT in patients with MM?

    18F-FDG PET/CT is recommended to distinguish smoldering MM from active MM if a whole-body X-ray is negative and a whole-body MRI is unavailable.

    18F-FDG PET/CT is of high value in the diagnosis and assessment of SP [2].

24. What are the patterns of 18F-FDG uptake in disease detection in symptomatic MM?

    1. Focal lesions (FLs): 18F-FDG uptake is greater than background (acquired on two successive images), either with or without bone osteolysis. Para medullary disease (PMD) and diffuse BM involvement-soft-tissue lesions are contiguous with bone involvement and with variable glucose metabolism and maximum standardized uptake values (SUVmax) [19–21, 28–30]. EMD is abnormal soft tissue without contiguous bone involvement [25, 31].
    2. Diffuse BM involvement-diffuse glucose uptake in the axial skeleton (greater than liver uptake and either heterogeneous or homogenous), and the disease may extend to the periphery.

25. What are the Italian myeloma criteria for PET USe (IMPeTUs) Criteria for 18F-FDG PET/CT reporting in MM?

    The IMPeTUs interpretation criteria were proposed to standardize the interpretation of PET in MM. Deauville criteria (a 5-point standardized visual interpretation scale) are used to identify the number of FLs and to characterize the involvement of PMD, EMD, and diffuse BM disease [32].

26. What percentage of newly diagnosed MM (NDMM) patients are false negative on PET-CT?

   In general, approximately 10–20% of NDMM patients are 18F-FDG PET-CT "false negative" at baseline due to low hexokinase-2 expression [25, 31, 33, 34], and these patients cannot be monitored after therapy using 18F-FDG PET/CT imaging. WB-MRI has higher sensitivity than 18F-FDG PET/CT (91% vs. 70%).

27. What is the IMPeTUs Classification for therapy response assessment?

   Complete metabolic response: Uptake ≤ liver uptake (Deauville criteria 1–3) in the BM and previously involved FLs, PMD, and EMD (if applicable) [3].

   Partial metabolic response: Decrease in number and/or activity of BM and previously involved FLs, PMD, and EMD (if applicable) but with a persistent lesion(s) with uptake > liver activity (DS 4 or 5) [3].

   Stable metabolic response: No significant change in BM uptake, and previously involved FLs, PMD, and EMD (if applicable) compared with baseline [3].

   Progressive metabolic disease: New FLs, PMD, or EMD (if applicable) compared with baseline consistent with MM [3].

28. What is the role of 11C-choline/11F-choline in MM?

   18F-choline, a tracer of phospholipids in the cell membrane. 18F-choline has no physiological uptake in the brain, allowing optimal evaluation of the skull. PET/CT performed in patients with suspected relapsing or progressive MM revealed more lesions on 18F-choline than 18F-FDG secondary to the higher tumor to background ratio [35].

29. What is the role of 11C-methionine in MM?

   Methionine, labeled with C-11, is an amino acid PET tracer. The radiolabeled amino acids show rapid metabolic absorption and incorporation into newly synthesized immunoglobulins. C11-methionine has a higher sensitivity in detecting FLs and EMD and better correlation with tumor burden [36, 37].

30. What is the role of 68Ga-Pentixafor PET/CT in MM?

   Chemokine (C-X-C motif) receptor 4 (CXCR4) is a key factor for tumor growth and metastasis in several types of human cancer, including MM. CXCR4 activation has been shown to correlate with MM-related bone disease [38].

   68Ga-Pentixafor may represent a valuable molecular probe for non-invasive assessment of CXCR4 expressed by tumor cells. However, more extensive prospective trials are necessary to assess the potential of 68Ga-Pentixafor PET in MM imaging [39].

31. What is role of 18F-FDG PET-MRI in MM?

   Hybrid PET/MRI simultaneously acquires morphological, functional, and metabolic information. PET-MRI can detect bone, as well as potential extramedullary lesions and medullary compression, without irradiation. 18F-FDG PET/MRI might improve FL detection and initial staging in patients with MM and might also be able to diagnose and localize residual disease activity [40–42].

32. What is the role of 18F-FDG in disease detection in SP ?

    18F-FDG PET-CT detects additional lesions with greater sensitivity and specificity than PSMRI [3, 43]. Its sensitivity, specificity, and positive and negative predictive values are 98% and 93%, 99% and 94%, 93% and 84%, and 99% and 98%, respectively [3, 43].

33. What is the prognostic value of pre-treatment 18F-FDG PET-CT in symptomatic MM?

    Several 18F-FDG PET-CT characteristics have been identified as possible high-risk biomarkers and could be used to define high-risk NDMM patients. Studies in NDMM patients have demonstrated that baseline-derived PET parameters of > 3 FLs, an FL SUVmax > 4.2 and EMD were associated with poorer progression-free survival (PFS) and overall survival (OS) [25, 31, 44].

    Large FLs are a decisive, independent factor for poor prognosis in NDMM [45, 46].

34. What is the role of 18F-FDG PET-CT in therapy assessment and MRD (minimal residual disease in MM?

    Post-treatment 18F-FDG PET/CT is a strong prognostic tool:

    1. 18F-FDG PET-CT can distinguish between metabolically active MM lesions and inactive fibrous residual osteolytic lesions, with an earlier and higher rate of scan normalization than MRI after therapy initiation [16, 25, 47, 48]. Currently, 18F-FDG PET-CT is the preferred imaging technique to evaluate and monitor metabolic response to therapy in MM [5, 6, 16].
    2. A persistent positive 18F-FDG PET-CT generally predicts a less favorable outcome [16, 25, 49–52].
    3. IMWG and expert consensus recommend performing post-treatment 18F-FDG PET-CT as a complementary tool to MRD assessment to assess for active EMD [53–55].
    4. The combination of negative MRD and negative post-treatment 18F-FDG PET-CT scans confirms complete eradication of the tumor inside and outside the BM, which is associated with longer PFS [48].
    5. Post-treatment 18F-FDG PET-CT normalization is an independent factor predictive of better PFS and OS.
    6. Persistence of FLs with SUVmax >4.2 after induction and post-transplant was associated with a shorter time to progression [31, 49].
    7. 18F-FDG PET-CT may not be appropriate for assessment of metabolic response to therapy if the baseline 18F-FDG PET-CT is negative, which can occur in 10–20% of patients with NDMM.

35. What is the checklist of items to be reported on 18F-FDG PET-CT scans during or after therapy?

    1. Presence of increased diffuse BM uptake (if applicable) and intensity of BM uptake, that is, DS (not including uptake in FLs).

2. Number of 18F-FDG PET/CT positive FLs (n = 0, n = 1–3, n > 3, or n > 10), that is, medullary, paramedullary, and/or extramedullary, and comparison with baseline measurements. oDS of most avid FL.
3. SUVmax of the most avid FL.
4. Based on CT interpretation, independent of 18F-FDG uptake, the number and size of new osteolytic lesions and/or osteolytic lesions that have increased in size compared with baseline measurements. Similar assessment for paramedullary and extramedullary lesions (if applicable).
5. Presence of fractures, for example, ribs, vertebra, on CT.
6. After therapy initiation, the IMPeTUs Classification should be used for therapy response assessment.

36. What are the criteria for progressive disease as per IMWG?

1. Progressive disease is defined as the appearance of new osteolytic lesion(s).
2. ≥50% increase from nadir in the sum of the products of the maximal perpendicular diameters of >1 lesion, or ≥50% increase in the longest diameter of a previous lesion >1 cm in the short axis [54].
3. Unless there is disease progression, change in treatment cannot be recommended based on post-treatment imaging results only [4].

37. What is the IMWG expert consensus on the optimal sequence of post-treatment 18F-FDG PET/CT scans?

There is no expert consensus on the optimal sequence of post-treatment 18F-FDG PET/CT scans: interim PET (after induction), end-of-therapy PET (pre-maintenance) and/or during maintenance [53].

38. What is the role of 18F-FDG PET-CT in MM relapse detection?

The appearance of new plasmacytoma and/or osteolytic bone lesion is one of the criteria defining relapse (or refractory MM) [30]. Imaging using 18F-FDG PET-CT is optional; however, it might be of interest for distinguishing between active and non-active (non-viable) MM FLs and for detecting EMD, which is more prevalent at relapse and adversely affects both time to progression and OS [16, 56–58].

39. What is the role 18F-FDG PET-CT in follow-up patients with MM?

1. The IMWG recommends yearly follow-up using 18F-FDG PET/CT in patients with a positive post-treatment 18F-FDG PET-CT who are at higher risk of early progression [16, 25, 49–52].
2. When MRD status is available, the EHA-ESMO Clinical Practice Guidelines recommend yearly follow-up 18F-FDG PET-CT in BM MRD-negative patients to confirm extramedullary MRD negativity. CT or MRI are recommended when symptomatic [56]. The same imaging technique should be used at each follow-up stage to enable comparison [3].
3. For SMM, 18F-FDG PET-CT can be used if the MRI is not feasible [3].

40. Should 18F-FDG PET-CT in staging scan report include variables?

Yes, an Should 18F-FDG PET-CT report for multiple myeloma (MM) staging should include variables to assess the extent of disease and predict outcomes

1. Metabolic state of the BM, including hypermetabolism in ribs and limbs, defined as homogenous or heterogeneous diffuse uptake of the pelvic spinal-peripheral skeleton liver uptake [1, 2, 53, 56].
2. Number and site of FLs on PET, with or without osteolysis on CT. An FL is defined as a visually detectable focal increase in 18F-FDG uptake surrounding BM uptake located in the skeleton (excluding sites of physiological tracer uptake) on two or more adjacent images, with or without osteolysis on CT.
3. The presence of PMD is defined as soft tissue extension contiguous with bone involvement.
4. The presence and site of EMD are defined as abnormal soft tissue without contiguous bone involvement.
5. Presence of fractures on CT.

41. Should 18F-FDG PET-CT scan report during or after treatment for therapy response assessment include variables?

Yes, an 18F-FDG PET-CT report for multiple myeloma (MM) staging should include variables to assess the scan report during or after treatment for therapy response assessment.

1. Complete metabolic response: Uptake $\leq$ liver uptake (DS 1–3) in the BM and previously involved FLs, PMD and EMD (if applicable) [1, 2, 53, 56].
2. Partial metabolic response: Decrease in number and/or uptake in BM and previously involved FLs, PMD and EMD (if applicable) but with persistent lesions with uptake liver uptake (DS 4 or 5).
3. Stable metabolic disease: No significant change in uptake in BM and previously involved FLs, PMD, and EMD (if applicable) compared with baseline.
4. Progressive metabolic disease: New FLs, PMD or EMD compared with baseline consistent with MM.

42. What are the interpretation issues/pitfalls of 18F-FDG PET-CT in MM?

1. Patients with anemia may manifest an increase in BM uptake ON FDG scan, reflecting a compensatory mechanism. However, a diffuse increase in BM uptake reduces contrast resolution on PET and the ability to detect coexistent FLs. In addition, it makes it difficult to differentiate from diffuse BM infiltration [1, 2, 53, 56].
2. Approximately 10–20% of patients have absent 18F-FDG uptake at staging despite histological confirmation of BM infiltration and/or osteolytic lesions on CT.
3. Sensitivity of 18F-FDG PET-CT is variable. Interpretation of a single post-therapy 18F-FDG PET-CT examination in the absence of baseline 18F-FDG PET-CT examination could lead to inaccurate assessment response to therapy [1, 2, 53, 56].

4. Interpreting early focal BM uptake without osteolysis on CT is difficult, particularly in those with low glucose metabolism or anemia.
5. False-positive 18F-FDG uptake can be seen in recent bone fractures and degenerative changes.
6. Osteosynthetic material could degrade image quality. It could result in false-positive uptake at the bone–osteosynthetic material interface, which might be related to ongoing bone healing or possibly bone infection [1, 2, 53, 56–58].
7. Differentiation of EMD from an unrelated non-malignant pathology, for example, inflammation, can be difficult, and in cases of uncertainty, targeted imaging or biopsy should be considered [1, 2, 53, 56–58].

References

1. Nanni C, Deroose CM, Balogova S, et al. EANM guidelines on the use of [^{18}F]FDG PET/CT in diagnosis, staging, prognostication, therapy assessment, and restaging of plasma cell disorders. Eur J Nucl Med Mol Imaging. 2024;52(1):171–92.
2. Cavo M, Terpos E, Nanni C, Moreau P, et al. Role of 18F-FDG PET/CT in the diagnosis and management of multiple myeloma and other plasma cell disorders: a consensus statement by the International Myeloma Working Group. Lancet Oncol. 2017;18(4):e206–17.
3. Rajkumar SV, Dimopoulos MA, Palumbo A, et al. International Myeloma Working Group updated criteria for the diagnosis of multiple myeloma. Lancet Oncol. 2014;15(12):e538–48.
4. Rajkumar SV. Updated diagnostic criteria and staging system for multiple myeloma. Am Soc Clin Oncol Educ Book. 2016;35:e418–23.
5. Hillengass J, Usmani S, Rajkumar SV, et al. International myeloma working group consensus recommendations on imaging in monoclonal plasma cell disorders. Lancet Oncol. 2019;20:e302–12.
6. Moreau P, San Miguel J, Sonneveld PR, Dimopoulos MA, Ludwig H, Einsele H, Zweegman S, Facon T, Cavo M, Terpos E, Goldschmidt H, Attal M, Buske C, et al. Multiple myeloma: ESMO clinical practice guidelines for diagnosis, treatment and follow-up. 2017. https://doi.org/10.1093/annonc/mdx096.
7. Healy CF, Murray JG, Eustace SJ, Madewell J, O'Gorman PJ, O'Sullivan P. Multiple myeloma: a review of imaging features and radiological techniques. Bone Marrow Res. 2011;2011:583439.
8. Durie BGM, Salmon SE. A clinical staging system for multiple myeloma. Correlation of measured myeloma cell mass with presenting clinical features, response to treatment, and survival. Cancer. 1975;36(3):842–54.
9. Baur-Melnyk A, Buhmann S, Becker C, et al. Whole-body MRI versus whole-body MDCT for staging of multiple myeloma. Am J Roentgenol. 2008;190(4):1097–104.
10. Lütje S, Rooy JWJ, Croockewit S, Koedam E, Oyen WJG, Raymakers RA. Role of radiography, MRI and FDG-PET/CT in diagnosing, staging and therapeutical evaluation of patients with multiple myeloma. Ann Hematol. 2009;88(12):1161–8.
11. Mahnken AH, Wildberger JE, Gehbauer G, et al. Multidetector CT of the spine in multiple myeloma: comparison with MR imaging and radiography. Am J Roentgenol. 2002;178(6):1429–36.
12. Avva R, Vanhemert RL, Barlogie B, Munshi N, Angtuaco EJ. CT-guided biopsy of focal lesions in patients with multiple myeloma may reveal new and more aggressive cytogenetic abnormalities. Am J Neuroradiol. 2001;22(4):781–5.
13. Baur-Melnyk A, Buhmann S, Dürr HR, Reiser M. Role of MRI for the diagnosis and prognosis of multiple myeloma. Eur J Radiol. 2005;55(1):56–63.

14. Vogler JB III, Murphy WA. Bone marrow imaging. Radiology. 1988;168(3):679–93.
15. Moulopoulos LA, Dimopoulos MA, Weber D, Fuller L, Libshitz HI, Alexanian R. Magnetic resonance imaging in the staging of solitary plasmacytoma of bone. J Clin Oncol. 1993;11(7):1311–5.
16. Cavo M, Terpos E, Nanni C, et al. Role of 18F-FDG PET/CT in the diagnosis and management of multiple myeloma and other plasma cell disorders: a consensus statement by the International Myeloma Working Group. 2017. https://doi.org/10.1016/S1470-2045(17)30189-4.
17. Dammacco F, Rubini G, Ferrari C, Vacca A, Racanelli V. 18F-FDG PET/CT: a review of diagnostic and prognostic features in multiple myeloma and related disorders. Clin Exp Med. 2015;15(1):1–18. https://doi.org/10.1007/s10238-014-0308-3.
18. Bailly C, Leforestier R, Jamet B, Carlier T, Bourgeois M, Guérard F, Touzeau C, Moreau P, Chérel M, Kraeber-Bodéré F, Bodet-Milin C. PET imaging for initial staging and therapy assessment in multiple myeloma patients. Int J Mol Sci. 2017;18(2):445.
19. Weng W, Dong M, Zhang J, et al. A systematic review of MRI, scintigraphy, FDG-PET and PET/CT for Diagnosis of multiple myeloma related bone disease – which is best? 2014. https://doi.org/10.7314/APJCP.2014.15.22.9879.
20. Lu Y, Chen J, Lin W, et al. FDG PET or PET/CT for detecting intramedullary and extramedullary lesions in multiple myeloma: a systematic review and meta-analysis. 2012. https://doi.org/10.1097/RLU.0b013e31825b2071.
21. Walker RC, Brown TL, Jones-Jackson LB, De Blanche L, Bartel T. Imaging of multiple myeloma and related plasma cell dyscrasias. 2012. https://doi.org/10.2967/jnumed.111.098830.
22. van Lammeren-Venema D, Regelink JC, Riphagen RI, Zweegman S, Hoekstra OS, Zijlstra JM. (1)(8)F-fluoro-deoxyglucose positron emission tomography in assessment of myeloma-related bone disease: a systematic review. Cancer. 2012;118(8):1971–81.
23. Lu YY, Chen J-H, Lin W-Y, Liang J-A, Wang H-Y, Tsai S-C, et al. FDG PET or PET/CT for detecting intramedullary and extramedullary lesions in multiple myeloma: a systematic review and meta-analysis. Clin Nucl Med. 2012;37(9):833–7.
24. Matteucci F, Paganelli G, Martinelli G, Cerchione C. PET/CT in multiple myeloma: beyond FDG. Front Oncol. 2021;25:10.
25. Moreau P, Attal M, Caillot D, et al. Prospective evaluation of magnetic resonance imaging and [18F] Fluorodeoxyglucose positron emission tomography-computed tomography at diagnosis and before maintenance therapy in symptomatic patients with multiple myeloma included in the IFM/DFCI 2009 trial: results of the IMAJEM study. J Clin Oncol. 2017;35(25):2911–8. https://doi.org/10.1200/JCO.2017.72.2975.
26. Zamagni E, Nanni C, Patriarca F, et al. A prospective comparison of 18F-fluorodeoxyglucose positron emission tomography-computed tomography, magnetic resonance imaging and whole-body planar radiographs in the assessment of bone disease in newly diagnosed multiple myeloma. 2007. https://doi.org/10.3324/haematol.10554.
27. Fonti R, Pace L, Cerchione C, et al. 18F-FDG PET/CT, 99mTc-MIBI, and MRI in the prediction of outcome of patients with multiple myeloma: a comparative study. 2015. https://doi.org/10.1097/RLU.0000000000000696.
28. Sager S, Ergül N, Ciftci H, Cetin G, Güner Sİ, Cermik TF. The value of FDG PET/CT in the initial staging and bone marrow involvement of patients with multiple myeloma. Skeletal Radiol. 2011;40 https://doi.org/10.1007/s00256-010-1088-9.
29. Mesguich C, Fardanesh R, Tanenbaum L, Chari A, Jagannath S, Kostakoglu L. State of the art imaging of multiple myeloma: Comparative review of FDG PET/CT imaging in various clinical settings. 2014. https://doi.org/10.1016/j.ejrad.2014.09.012.
30. Kraeber-Bodéré F, Zweegman S, Perrot A, Hulin C, et al. Prognostic value of positron emission tomography/computed tomography in transplanteligible newly diagnosed multiple myeloma patients from CASSIOPEIA: the CASSIOPET study. 2023. https://doi.org/10.3324/haematol.2021.280051.
31. Zamagni E, Patriarca F, Nanni C, et al. Prognostic relevance of 18-F FDG PET/CT in newly diagnosed multiple myeloma patients treated with up-front autologous transplantation. 2011. https://doi.org/10.1182/blood-2011-06-361386.

32. Nanni C, Versari A, Chauvie S, et al. Interpretation criteria for FDG PET/CT in multiple myeloma (IMPeTUs): final results. IMPeTUs (Italian myeloma criteria for PET USe). Eur J Nucl Med Mol Imaging. 2018;45 https://doi.org/10.1007/s00259-017-3909-8.

33. Rasche L, Angtuaco E, McDonald JE, et al. Low expression of hexokinase-2 is associated with false-negative FDG–positron emission tomography in multiple myeloma. 2017. https://doi.org/10.1182/blood-2017-03-774422.

34. Alberge J, Kraeber-Bodéré F, Jamet B, et al. Molecular signature of 18F-FDG PET biomarkers in newly diagnosed multiple myeloma patients: a genome-wide transcriptome analysis from the CASSIOPET study. 2022. https://doi.org/10.2967/jnumed.121.262884.

35. Mesguich C, Hulin C, Lascaux A, Bordenave L, Marit G, Hindié E. Choline PET/CT in multiple myeloma. Cancers (Basel). 2020;12(6):1394.

36. Hemrom A, Tupalli A, Alavi A, Kumar R. 18F-FDG versus non-FDG PET tracers in multiple myeloma. PET Clin. 2022;17:415–30.

37. Matteucci F, Paganelli G, Martinelli G, Cerchione C. PET/CT in multiple myeloma: beyond FDG. Front Oncol. 2021;25:622501.

38. Lapa C, Schreder M, Schirbel A. [68Ga]Pentixafor-PET/CT for imaging of chemokine receptor CXCR4 expression in multiple myeloma – comparison to [18F]FDG and laboratory values. Theranostics. 2017;7(1):205–12.

39. Wang M, Zhang J, Liu L, et al. The role of 68Ga-Pentixafor PET in multiple myeloma. Clin Translat Imaging. 2023;11:453–63.

40. Garderet L, Kharroubi-Lakouas D, Weil D, et al. The role of PET-MRI in multiple myeloma patients. Blood. 2020;136(1):12.

41. Mulé S, Reizine E, Blanc-Durand P, Baranes L, Zerbib P, Burns R, Nouri R, Itti E, Luciani A. Whole-body functional MRI and PET/MRI in multiple myeloma. Cancer. 2020;12:3155.

42. Burns R, Mule S, Zerbib P, et al. Whole-Body Functional PET-MR for Multiple Myeloma Staging: Impact of Sequence Design on Bone Marrow Infiltration and Focal Lesion Assessment. In Proceedings of the Radiological Society of North America 2018 Scientific Assembly and Annual Meeting, Chicago, IL, USA, 20–30 November 2018.

43. Salaun P, Gastinne T, Frampas E, Bodet-Milin C, Moreau P, Bodéré-Kraeber F. FDG-positron-emission tomography for staging and therapeutic assessment in patients with plasmacytoma. 2008. https://doi.org/10.3324/haematol.12654.

44. Bartel TB, Haessler J, Brown TLY, et al. F18-fluorodeoxyglucose positron emission tomography in the context of other imaging techniques and prognostic factors in multiple myeloma. 2009. https://doi.org/10.1182/blood-2009-03-213280.

45. Rasche L, Chavan SS, Stephens OW, et al. Spatial genomic heterogeneity in multiple myeloma revealed by multi-region sequencing. 2017. https://doi.org/10.1038/s41467-017-00296-y

46. Rasche L, Angtuaco EJ, Alpe TL, et al. The presence of large focal lesions is a strong independent prognostic factor in multiple myeloma. 2018. https://doi.org/10.1182/blood-2018-04-842880.

47. Rama S, Suh CH, Kim KW, Durieux JC, Ramaiya NH, Tirumani SH. Comparative performance of whole-body MRI and FDG PET/CT in evaluation of multiple myeloma treatment response: systematic review and meta-analysis. 2022. https://doi.org/10.2214/AJR.21.26381.

48. Rasche L, Alapat D, Kumar M, et al. Combination of flow cytometry and functional imaging for monitoring of residual disease in myeloma. 2019. https://doi.org/10.1038/s41375-018-0329-0.

49. Zamagni E, Nanni C, Mancuso K, et al. PET/CT improves the definition of complete response and allows to detect otherwise unidentifiable skeletal progression in multiple myeloma. 2015. https://doi.org/10.1158/1078-0432.CCR-15-0396.

50. Zamagni E, Nanni C, Dozza L, et al. Standardization of 18 F-FDG–PET/CT according to deauville criteria for metabolic complete response definition in newly diagnosed multiple myeloma. 2021. https://doi.org/10.1200/jco.20.00386.

51. Davies FE, Rosenthal A, Rasche L, et al. Treatment to suppression of focal lesions on positron emission tomography-computed tomography is a therapeutic goal in newly diagnosed multiple myeloma. 2018. https://doi.org/10.3324/haematol.2017.177139.

52. Zamagni E, Oliva S, Gay F et al. Impact of minimal residual disease standardised assessment by FDG-PET/CT in transplant-eligible patients with newly diagnosed multiple myeloma enrolled in the imaging sub-study of the FORTE trial. 2023. https://doi.org/10.1016/j.eclinm.2023.102017.
53. Nanni C, Kobe C, Baeßler B, et al. European Association of Nuclear Medicine (EANM) focus 4 consensus recommendations: molecular imaging and therapy in haematological tumours. 2023. https://doi.org/10.1016/S2352-3026(23)00030-3.
54. Kumar S, Paiva B, Anderson KC, et al. International Myeloma Working Group consensus criteria for response and minimal residual disease assessment in multiple myeloma. 2016. https://doi.org/10.1016/S1470-2045(16)30206-6.
55. Costa LJ, Derman BA, Bal S, et al. International harmonization in performing and reporting minimal residual disease assessment in multiple myeloma trials. Leukemia. 2021;35 https://doi.org/10.1038/s41375-020-01012-4.
56. Zamagni E, Barbato S, Cavo M. How I treat high-risk multiple myeloma. Blood. 2022;139 https://doi.org/10.1182/blood.2020008733.
57. Dimopoulos MA, Moreau P, Terpos E, et al. Multiple myeloma: EHA-ESMO clinical practice guidelines for diagnosis, treatment and follow-up. 2021. https://doi.org/10.1097/HS9.0000000000000528.
58. Lapa C, Luckerath K, Malzahn U, et al. 18 FDG-PET/CT for prognostic stratification of patients with multiple myeloma relapse after stem cell transplantation. Oncotarget. 2014:10.18632/oncotarget.22.

Bone Tumors

1. What is the classification of bone tumors?

    Bone tumors are broadly classified based on the World Health Organization pathologic classification system as chondrogenic tumors, osteogenic tumors, fibrogenic tumors, vascular tumors, osteoclastic giant cell-rich tumors, notochordal tumors, other mesenchymal tumors of bone, and hematopoietic neoplasms [1, 2].

2. What are the primary malignant bone tumors?

    The primary malignant bone tumors include multiple myeloma, osteosarcoma, adamantinoma, chondrosarcoma, Ewing's sarcoma, fibrosarcoma, undifferentiated pleomorphic sarcoma, lymphoma of bone, and malignant giant cell tumor [1–4].

3. What are the benign bone tumors and cysts?

    Giant cell tumors of bone, osteoblastoma, chondroblastoma, chondromyxoid fibroma, enchondroma, non-ossifying fibromas, osteochondromas, and osteoid osteomas [1–4].

4. What are the metastatic bone tumors?

    Any cancer may metastasize to bone. However, metastases from carcinomas are the most common in patients with breast, prostate, lung, kidney, thyroid, and colon carcinomas [1–4].

5. What are the common positron emission tomography (PET) radiopharmaceuticals used in imaging bone tumors?

    PET radiopharmaceuticals in imaging bone tumors include ^{18}F-fluorodeoxyglucose (18F-FDG), bone-imaging agent sodium fluoride 18F-NaF, proliferation marker 18F-fluorodeoxythymidine, amino acid tracers (11C-methionine and 18F-fluoroethyltyrosine), and biomarkers of neoangiogenesis (18F-galacto-RGD) [5].

6. What is the role of conventional radiography in primary bone tumors?

   Radiographs provide information regarding the location, margins, matrix mineralization, periosteal reaction, and aggressiveness of the lesion [6–8].

7. What are the limitations of conventional radiography in primary bone tumors?

   Radiography is a valuable imaging modality for initial differential diagnosis of primary bone tumors. However, the limitations include (a) anatomic overlap can obscure abnormalities, (b) limited capacity to evaluate soft tissue, (c) limited assessment of extraosseous tumor volume, (d) relationship of the extraosseous tumor to surrounding structures, and (e) extent of disease in the intact marrow cavity [6–8].

8. What are the advantages of computed tomography (CT) in primary bone tumors?

   CT scan is useful in assessing cortical involvement and breakthrough. CT is useful in the assessment of tumors in complex-shaped bones (e.g., spine and pelvis) [6, 9–11].

9. What are the limitations of CT in primary bone tumors?

   The limitations of CT in primary bone tumors are in differentiating tumor invasion of the medullary cavity and reactive non-neoplastic loss of cancellous bone [8, 10, 11].

10. What are the advantages of magnetic resonance imaging (MRI) in primary bone tumors?

    MRI is useful in the assessment of the extent of tumor spread to detect tumor involvement of the adjacent muscle compartments, neurovascular structures, and joints [6, 9–11].

11. What are the limitations of MRI in primary bone tumors?

    MRI does not allow accurate malignant or benign lesion prediction based solely on its signal intensity [11]. MRI is superior to CT in assessing recurrent disease [11, 12].

12. What are the benign bone tumors exhibiting high FDG avidity?

    Benign bone tumors exhibiting high FDG avidity include giant cell tumors, chondroblastomas, osteoblastoma, osteoid osteomas, Langerhans cell histiocytosis, chondromyxoid fibromas, brown tumors, fibrous dysplasia, fibroxanthomas (non-ossifying fibromas), desmoplastic fibromas, and aneurysmal bone cysts [11, 13].

13. Which benign tumors exhibit typically low FDG avidity?

    Benign lesions with low FDG avidity included osteochondromas, enchondromas, hemangiomas, and intraosseous lipomas. In addition, low-grade osteosarcoma and Ewing sarcoma might show low FDG avidity [11–13].

14. What is the role of 18F-FDG PET/CT in staging primary bone tumors?

    The role of 18F-FDG PET/CT in the initial diagnostic work-up of bone tumors is still not well established. In patients with metastatic osteosarcoma and Ewing sarcoma, 18F-FDG PET/CT is reported to have higher sensitivity

(98% vs. 83%) and specificity (97% vs. 78%) than plain radiography for detecting distant metastases, apart from pulmonary nodules. In the detection of pulmonary nodules, 18F-FDG PET/CT was found to have a higher specificity (96% vs. 87%) but lower sensitivity (80% vs. 93%) than did conventional imaging [11, 14].

15. What is the spectrum of FDG uptake in primary bone tumors?

A spectrum of FDG uptake has been reported in primary bone tumors, with more aggressive lesions tending to be more FDG avid than nonaggressive lesions. Malignancies are generally significantly more avid than benign lesions [11].

16. What is the role of 18F-FDG PET-CT in assessing treatment response in bone tumors?

18F-FDG PET/CT is useful in the assessment of therapeutic response. Pre-therapeutic FDG uptake, post-therapeutic FDG uptake, and change in FDG uptake have been found to correlate with progression-free and overall survival in osteosarcoma. Post-therapeutic avidity was found to correlate with progression-free survival in Ewing sarcoma [11, 13, 14].

17. What is the role of 18F-FDG PET-CT in osteosarcoma?

18F-FDG PET/CT is useful for staging, detecting recurrence, and predicting histologic response and prognosis in investigating osteosarcoma. PET/CT showed 100% sensitivity [11, 13, 15] for detecting primary lesions. During staging, PET/CT is useful for differential diagnosis of primary bone neoplasms and for detecting metastatic lesions. Strobel et al. compared the diagnostic accuracy of plain radiography, PET, and PET/CT and found that FDG PET/CT showed 95% sensitivity and 77% specificity. Quartuccio et al. reported that FDG PET/CT has higher accuracy for detecting bone metastasis than CT or dedicated MRI [16].

18. What are the pooled sensitivity and specificity of 18F-FDG PET-CT in detecting lung metastases in osteosarcoma?

The pooled sensitivity and specificity for detecting lung metastases are 81% and 94%, respectively [13, 15].

19. What are the pooled sensitivity and specificity of 18F-FDG PET-CT in detecting bone metastases in osteosarcoma?

For detecting bone metastases in osteosarcoma, the pooled sensitivity is 93% and specificity is 97% [13, 15].

20. What is the role of 18F-FDG PET-CT in detecting recurrence in osteosarcoma?

18F-FDG PET/CT is useful in detecting osteosarcoma recurrence after completion of treatment. The pooled sensitivity and specificity are 91% and 93%, respectively [13, 15].

21. What is the role of 18F-FDG PET-CT in Ewing's sarcoma?

18F-FDG PET/CT is sensitive and accurate in diagnosing, staging, and detecting the recurrence of Ewing's sarcoma.

The reported sensitivity and specificity of 18F-FDG PET/CT in detecting total lesions are 93% and 74%. Notably, 97% and 68% were used to detect Ewing's sarcoma primary lesions, 76% and 92% for lung metastases, 84% and 93% for bone metastases, and 90% and 93% for recurrent disease [17].

22. What is the role of 18F-FDG PET-CT in chondrosarcoma?

The diagnostic accuracy of 18F-FDG PET/CT for chondrosarcoma is high, with a pooled sensitivity and specificity of 18F-FDG PET for diagnosing chondrosarcoma of 94% and 89%, respectively [18].

23. What is the role of 18F-FDG PET-CT in soft tissue sarcoma?

18F-FDG-PET-CT imaging has been used in soft tissue sarcomas to guide biopsy and assess therapeutic response, staging, follow-up, and prognosis [19]. 18F-FDG PET/CT is useful for the initial assessment of sarcomas and detecting their recurrences [20]. 18F-F-FDG PET/CT is useful in distinguishing malignant lesions from benign lesions in soft tissue sarcoma patients with different uptake patterns according to the histological type [21]. However, 18F-FDG PET has limited use in myxoid liposarcoma and synovial sarcoma, as these tumors often show a low uptake of glucose [22].

24. What is the role of PET/MRI in primary bone tumors?

18F-FDG-PET/MRI is useful in diagnosing and evaluating bone tumors in primary and metastatic settings. PET/MRI has advantages over PET/CT for its excellent soft tissue contrast and lower radiation exposure, a clear benefit for pediatric patients. PET/MRI showed a 73% reduction in radiation exposure compared with PET/CT and demonstrated an identical rate of detecting lesions [23–25]. PET/MRI can improve the monitoring of response to immunotherapy and potentially be used for the identification of non-responders by tumor-associated macrophage imaging using iron oxide nanoparticles [24].

25. What are the limitations of PET/MRI in primary bone tumors?

The typical limitations of PET/MRI include long acquisition time and false positives (e.g., trauma and osteomyelitis) [26].

26. What are the advantages of using 18F-FDG PET/CT in bone tumors?

18F-FDG PET/CT is useful for staging, detecting recurrence, and predicting treatment response and prognosis. 18F-FDG PET is useful for the detection of nodal and distant metastases [11].

27. What are the pitfalls to the Use of 18F-FDG PET/CT in bone tumors?

Metabolic activity is not accurate in differentiating benign and malignant tumors.

Post-surgical or post-radiation inflammatory changes might persist for several months to years following treatment and need to be considered when the operative bed is assessed. In addition, metal artifacts secondary to tumor prosthesis might impact lesion detectability and reader confidence [27].

28. What is the role of dual time point imaging in primary bone tumors?

In general, malignancies can progressively accumulate FDG for several hours, and background activity is continually cleared. The prolonged uptake periods often increase lesion detectability and higher measured tumor activity. Dual time point imaging in bone tumors is used to differentiate malignant from benign bone lesions using 1- and 2-h acquisition times. In general, FDG accumulation in malignancies tends to increase for several hours, and the FDG uptake of benign lesions typically undergoes an early plateau, which provides a potential means of differentiation [11, 28].

29. What are the sensitivity, specificity, and accuracy of dual time point PET imaging in bone tumors?

The sensitivity, specificity, and accuracy of PET using the standard 1-hour image acquisition time were 96%, 44%, and 72%, respectively. The sensitivity, specificity, and accuracy of PET using the delayed imaging technique, 2-h image acquisition time, were 91%, 76%, and 84%, respectively [11, 28, 29].

30. What are the limitations of dual time point imaging?

Routine use of dual time point imaging may not be practical because of prolonged scheduling time requirements, and there is no consensus on the timing of delayed imaging or the threshold value of FDG uptake for discriminating between malignant and benign lesions [11, 28, 29].

References

1. Choi JH, Ro JY. The 2020 WHO classification of tumors of bone: an updated review. Adv Anat Pathol. 2021;28(3):119.
2. Joyce MJ, Joyce DM. MDS manual professional version, overview of bone and joint tumours. www.mdsmanuals.com.
3. Weber K, Damron TA, Frassica FJ, Sim FH. Malignant bone tumors. Instr Course Lect. 2008;57:673–88.
4. Rozeman LB, Cleton-Jansen AM, Hogendoorn PC. Pathology of primary malignant bone and cartilage tumours. Int Orthop. 2006;30(6):437–44.
5. Wieder HA, Pomykala KL, Benz MR, Buck AK, Herrmann K. PET tracers in musculoskeletal disease beyond FDG. Semin Musculoskelet Radiol. 2014;18(2):123–32.
6. Costelloe CM, Madewell JE. Radiography in the initial diagnosis of primary bone tumors. AJR Am J Roentgenol. 2013;200(1):3–7.
7. Nomikos GC, Murphey MD, Kransdorf MJ, Bancroft LW, Peterson JJ. Primary bone tumors of the lower extremities. Radiol Clin North Am. 2002;40:971–90.
8. Resnick D, Greenway GD. Tumors and tumor-like lesions of bone: imaging and pathology of specific lesions. In: Resnick D, editor. Bone and joint imaging. 2nd ed. Philadelphia: W.B. Saunders; 1996. p. 991–1065.
9. Peh WC. The role of imaging in the staging of bone tumors. Crit Rev Oncol Hematol. 1999;31:147–67.
10. Teo HE, Peh WC. Primary bone tumors of adulthood. Cancer Imaging. 2004;4(2):74–83.
11. Costelloe CM, Chuang HH, Madewell JE. FDG PET/CT of primary bone tumors. AJR Am J Roentgenol. 2014;202(6):W521–31.

12. Nascimento D, Suchard G, Hatem M, de Abreu A. The role of magnetic resonance imaging in the evaluation of bone tumours and tumour-like lesions. Insights Imaging. 2014 Aug;5(4):419–40.
13. Oh C, Bishop MW, Cho SY, Im HJ, Shulkin BL. ^{18}F-FDG PET/CT in the Management of Osteosarcoma. J Nucl Med. 2023;64(6):842–51.
14. London K, Stege C, Cross S, et al. ^{18}F-FDG PET/CT compared to conventional imaging modalities in pediatric primary bone tumors. Pediatr Radiol. 2012;42:418–30.
15. Liu F, Zhang Q, Zhou D, Dong J. Effectiveness of ^{18}F-FDG PET/CT in the diagnosis and staging of osteosarcoma: a meta-analysis of 26 studies. BMC Cancer. 2019;19:323.
16. Quartuccio N, Fox J, Kuk D, et al. Pediatric bone sarcoma: diagnostic performance of ^{18}F-FDG PET/CT versus conventional imaging for initial staging and follow-up. AJR. 2015;204:153–60.
17. Seth N, Seth I, Bulloch G, Siu AHY, Guo A, Chatterjee R, MacManus M, Donnan L. [18] F-FDG PET and PET/CT as a diagnostic method for Ewing sarcoma: a systematic review and meta-analysis. Pediatr Blood Cancer. 2022;69(3):e29415.
18. Zhang Q, Xi Y, Li D, Yuan Z, Dong J. The utility of ^{18}F-FDG PET and PET/CT in the diagnosis and staging of chondrosarcoma: a meta-analysis. J Orthop Surg Res. 2020;22;15(1):229.
19. Kassem TW, Abdelaziz O, Emad-Eldin S. Diagnostic value of 18F-FDG-PET/CT for the follow-up and restaging of soft tissue sarcomas in adults. Diagn Interv Imaging. 2017;98(10):693–8.
20. Charest M, Hickeson M, Lisbona R, Novales-Diaz JA, Derbekyan V, Turcotte RE. FDG PET/CT imaging in primary osseous and soft tissue sarcomas: a retrospective review of 212 cases. Eur J Nucl Med Mol Imaging. 2009;36(12):1944–51.
21. Nose H, Otsuka H, Otomi Y, Terazawa K, Takao S, Iwamoto S, Harada M. Correlations between F-18 FDG PET/CT and pathological findings in soft tissue lesions. J Med Investig. 2013;60(3–4):184–90.
22. Sambri A, Bianchi G, Longhi A, Righi A, Donati DM, Nanni C, Fanti S, Errani C. The role of 18F-FDG PET/CT in soft tissue sarcoma. Nucl Med Commun. 2019 Jun;40(6):626–31.
23. Schäfer JF, Gatidis S, Schmidt H, et al. Simultaneous whole-body PET/MR imaging in comparison to PET/CT in pediatric oncology: initial results. Radiology. 2014;273:220–31.
24. Baratto L, Hawk KE, States L, et al. PET/MRI improves management of children with cancer. J Nucl Med. 2021;62:1334–40.
25. Behzadi AH, Raza SI, Carrino JA, et al. Applications of PET/CT and PET/MR imaging in primary bone malignancies. PET Clin. 2018;13(4):623–34.
26. Padwal J, Baratto L, Chakraborty A, Hawk K, Spunt S, Avedian R, Daldrup-Link HE. PET/MR of pediatric bone tumors: what the radiologist needs to know. Skeletal Radiol. 2022;52(3):315–28.
27. Benz MR, Crompton JG, Harder D. PET/CT variants and pitfalls in bone and soft tissue sarcoma. Semin Nucl Med. 2021;51(6):584–92.
28. Tian R, Su M, Tian Y, et al. Dual-time point PET/CT with F-18 FDG for the differentiation of malignant and benign bone lesions. Skeletal Radiol. 2009;38:451–8.
29. Schillaci O. Use of dual-point fluorodeoxyglucose imaging to enhance sensitivity and specificity. Semin Nucl Med. 2012;42:267–80.

Radiotherapy Planning

25

1. What is radiotherapy (RT)?

    The delivery of ionizing radiation to achieve cell kill and tumor shrinkage in cancer. The success or failure is determined by the 4R principle in radiobiology: repair of DNA damage, redistribution of cells in the cell cycle, repopulation, and reoxygenation of hypoxic tumor areas [1].

2. What are the different RT treatment intents?

    - Curative "radical" treatment
    - In combination with surgery (pre-op RT: neoadjuvant, post-op RT: adjuvant therapy)
    - In combination with radiosensitizing agents such as chemotherapy and targeted treatment
    - Palliative treatment

3. What is the goal of RT planning?

    RT planning aims to produce a dose distribution within the patient that will destroy the tumor while sparing as much healthy tissue as possible.

4. What is the different external beam radiotherapy (EBRT) delivery techniques? [2]

    (a) Conventional (2D) radiation therapy: a single beam from one to four directions.

    (b) 3D conformal radiation therapy: this is a 3D technique that delivers the highest possible dose of radiation to the tumor while sparing healthy tissue. It requires CT planning and considers axial anatomy and complex tissue contours.

    (c) Intensity-modulated radiation therapy (IMRT): this technique is an advanced form of 3D conformal RT, which allows higher and varying doses of radiation to the tumor through modulation of each beam intensity and planning to one or more high-intensity radiation areas and any number of

S. Raja et al., *Question and Answers in PET/CT*, https://doi.org/10.1007/978-3-032-00821-3_25

lower intensity areas within the same field. Overall, IMRT allows greater control of dose distribution within the target.

(d) Stereotactic radiosurgery (treatments to brain or spine) and stereotactic body radiotherapy/stereotactic ablative radiotherapy utilize 3D coordinates to maximize treatment precision with smaller margins and higher dose, usually to irradiate a small volume (<4 cm) in one fraction. Delivery systems include IMRT linear accelerators, Gamma Knife, or CyberKnife.

(e) Particle therapy. The most common type is proton-beam therapy, where higher dose gradients can be delivered while reducing the dose to adjacent organs at risk. Its application is in tumors close to critical organs, such as the brain and spine. Carbon ion therapy is another type of particle therapy, but it has limited worldwide availability.

5. How is EBRT delivered?

   EBRT is delivered by a medical linear accelerator.

6. What is the role of positron emission tomography (PET)-computed tomography (CT) in RT treatment planning?

   While CT is the best modality for RT planning in terms of dosimetry and spatial resolution, PET allows accurate tumor delineation and co-registration on CT images. CT for co-registration can be acquired either from a separate CT scanner or by obtaining images on an integrated PET-CT unit while the patient is in the treatment position [3, 4].

7. What are the benefits of PET-CT in RT treatment planning?

   • Integrated planning PET-CT machines reduce intra-observer and inter-observer variation in tumor delineation and allow better assessment of anatomical gross tumor volume (GTV) and biological target volume through functional sub-volumes [5].
   • Inhomogeneous dose distribution can be applied to the target volume (dose escalation and dose redistribution), depending on regions of radioresistance or risk of radiation-induced toxicity; this concept is called "dose painting" [4–6].
   • Increased accuracy of target volume delineation. GTV delineated from 18F-FDG PET was found to be the closest to the pathological GTV from surgical specimens and significantly smaller than GTV delineated by CT and MRI in pharyngolaryngeal SCC [7, 8].
   • Separate RT planning CT hospital visits are no longer required.
   • Errors associated with acquiring and registering images at different time points are removed.
   • The use of a flat coach minimizes the variation in co-registration of non-dedicated diagnostic PET-CT and planning CT.
   • Availability of motion management techniques such as respiratory gating [9].
   • When compared to CT-based RT planning in non-small cell lung cancer (NSCLC), there is strong evidence of [10]:

  - More accurate estimate of gross tumor through the identification of unde-
    tected nodal involvement on CT and exclusion of PET-negative but
    enlarged lymph nodes
  - Ability to demarcate the border between tumor and collapsed lung in the
    presence of atelectasis
  - Resultant change in tumor contour and RT treatment plan
  - Avoidance of geographic miss or sparing of large volumes of normal tissue

8. What are the disadvantages of PET-CT in RT treatment planning?

   - Disadvantages of individual radiopharmaceuticals for PET imaging. For
     instance, 18F-FDG is not specific for malignant processes and is taken up by
     processes with increased glucose turnover, such as infection and inflammation
   - Scanner bore size can limit patient eligibility
   - Cost of additional software, hardware, and gating device staff training
   - Development of a dedicated protocol, including a different (non-attenuation
     correction low-dose CT) CT acquisition protocol in direct planning
   - Presence of RT staff during PET-CT setup, patient positioning, and
     acquisition
   - Patient discomfort due to the use of flat couch overlay and immobilization
     device, in RT planning patient positioning
   - RT planner specialist expertise
   - Input from Medical Physics Experts from both PET and RT departments to
     set up quality control requirements, radiation dose assessments, and safety
     considerations
   - Cost of data storage, data transfer solutions, and a compatible treatment
     planning system
   - Limited automated segmentation algorithms [9, 11]
   - Spatial resolution of PET: small lesions may not be detected if the tracer is
     not intensely avid. The margins of a lesion can appear fuzzy and indistinct
   - Longer appointment time slot
   - Suboptimal co-registration of PET and CT due to involuntary and involun-
     tary patient movement and internal organ movement
   - Variability in functional image interpretation, such as windowing, color
     scale, and thresholding, can affect GTV delineation
   - Inter-observation variation if a standardized software-based contouring pro-
     tocol is not used [10]

9. What is direct and indirect RT planning?
   Direct planning: The CT component of the PET-CT is used to co-register the
   PET component to delineate target/healthy tissue in RT treatment planning.
   A separate RT planning CT is not required.
   Indirect planning: A separate RT planning CT is acquired and registered
   with the RT planning PET-CT, which is more accurate [11].

10. What are the registration techniques in RT treatment planning?
    (a) Rigid registration is a linear transformation that includes translation and rotation only, preserving the distances between all points in the image.
    (b) Affine registration is also linear, but, in addition to translation and rotation, it includes scaling, shearing, and plane reflection. Distances between points in the image are not preserved, but parallel lines remain parallel.
    (c) Deformable registration is a non-linear transformation and maps points from one image to another [11].

11. What are the methods of volume delineation?

    1. Manual segmentation performed by a clinical oncologist and nuclear medicine physician/radiologist
    2. Automated segmentation algorithms are split into two broad groups:

       • Simple threshold-based techniques (fixed or adaptive)
       • More advanced algorithms but few are widely available, and most are not fully validated [11].

12. What are the common tumor groups utilizing PET-CT in RT treatment planning?

    • Brain
    • Head and neck
    • Lung (NSCLC and small cell lung cancer (SCLC))
    • Esophageal, gastric, colorectal, and anal malignancies
    • Prostate
    • Gynecological malignancies
    • Pediatrics—Hodgkin's lymphoma, nasopharyngeal carcinoma, solid tumors such as bone and soft tissue sarcomas, Wilm's tumor, and neuroblastomas

13. What are the special patient considerations in PET-CT RT planning?
    Patient positioning and immobilization are vital in successful RT planning.
    Special considerations should be considered, addressed, and controlled, including [10, 11]:

    • General health—does the patient suffer from pain, dyspnea, coughing, nausea, agitation, anxiety, involuntary movements, or claustrophobia? Is there a history of learning disability, dementia, or acute confusion? Is there a need for a translator, carer, or comforter?
    • Age—young children may require anesthesia.
    • Weight—camera weight limit and gantry bore diameter.
    • Respiration and organ motion (e.g., gastric, intestinal, and urinary bladder distension) can alter the positioning of the target.
    • Clothing—variation in clothing may affect target positioning.
    • Underlays such as blankets and sheets between the camera and treatment planning equipment.
    • Overlay/couch top bending or flexing, creating different geometry

- Laser light—alignment variation between the scanner and treatment equipment.
- Certain treatment areas are challenging to immobilze.
- Fixation device should be standardized.
- Placement of fixation devices should be standardized.
- Skin markers disappearing or becoming indistinct/tattoos from previous treatment planning can add to the confusion and increase the risk of mistakes.
- Staff experience and skills.
- Environment—temperature, lighting, noise, patient comfort, and rapport with staff.
- Disease progression—progression between planning PET-CT and the first RT session may render planning inaccurate.
- Preparation for different tumor groups—gastric and urinary bladder distention requirements may dictate the consumption of fluid during uptake time and separate image acquisition.
- Patient position of specific treatment—supine versus prone, arms up versus down.
- Previous PET-CTs—after baseline studies should be performed on the same scanner, with the same patient preparation and positioning and acquisition.

14. What are the special equipment considerations in PET-CT RT planning? [11, 12]
    - Intravenous contrast injector, equipment, and contrast administration protocols
    - PET-CT camera gantry. An extra-large gantry opening is desired to allow the placement of arms above the head if required.
    - Flat bed/couch overlay/CT overlay—a flat carbon fiber CT overlay must replace the standard couch overlay to allow the same geometry as the RT couch top.
    - Immobilization device. Placed on the CT overlay and treatment couch, this device is a standardized positioning and fixation system that includes pads and smaller accessories. The device should be made of a material that gives minimal attenuation for imaging and no interference with the skin-sparing benefits of a high-voltage linear accelerator—for example, thermoplastic masks for head and neck treatments, breast boards for thoracic and upper abdominal region, and belly boards for prone positioning planning.
    - Padding or special body part cushions (e.g., head or foot rests and knee fix cushions) to enhance patient comfort in non-target areas.
    - External laser system. The coordinate system uses three axes for treatment setup and marking of external reference points on the patient's skin and any immobilization device.
    - Skin mark drawings of reference isocenter as indicated by laser. This needs to align with the internal scanner laser:

- Metal pins or wires placed on the patient to define isocenter on CT
- Patient bell
- Visual and audio surveillance
- Software for imaging analysis, including PET volume contouring and image quantification
- Connection with planning system (direct or remote transfer) and data storage solutions
- Regular quality control program for the PET-CT camera and the external laser system for alignment

15. What is "isocenter" in RT planning?

    The isocenter refers to the center of gantry rotation and the RT linear accelerator. This allows the patient to be in the same position for all the treatment fields [12].

16. How is the planning target volume (PTV) generated?

    PTV includes macroscopic tumor tissue (GTV), the putative microscopic invasion (clinical tumor volume, CTV), and a safety margin that depends on the radiation technique and precise patient placement [11, 13] (Fig. 25.1).

17. What additional volumes and regions are considered in dose planning?

    A radiation oncologist marks the internal target volume and takes into account the movement of the tumor within the body. Organs at risk are healthy tissues/organs such as eyes, spinal cord, and kidneys and should be placed near the CTV.

18. What is the cost-effectiveness of PET-CT in RT planning?

    18F-FDG PET-based RT planning in NSCLC nodal irradiation is cost-effective compared to CT-based planning [14].

    A prospective pilot study found DOTATATE PET/MRI to be more cost-effective than MRI alone in treatment planning of recurrent benign and malignant (intermediate risk) meningiomas [15]. A larger cost–benefit analysis and outcome data are awaited.

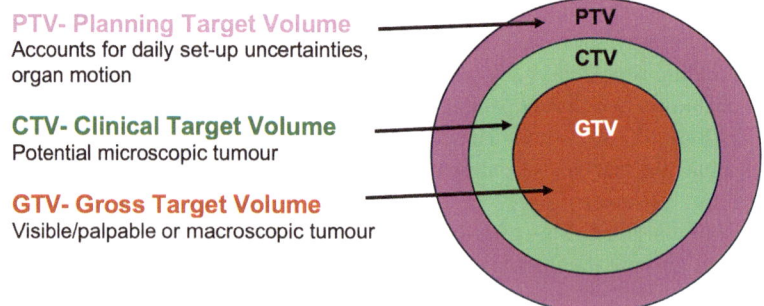

PTV- Planning Target Volume
Accounts for daily set-up uncertainties, organ motion

CTV- Clinical Target Volume
Potential microscopic tumour

GTV- Gross Target Volume
Visible/palpable or macroscopic tumour

Fig. 25.1 Pictorial description of GTV, CTV, and PTV

References

1. Pajonk F, Vlashi E, McBride WH. Radiation resistance of cancer stem cells: the 4 R's of radio-biology revisited. Stem Cells. 2010;28(4):639–48. https://doi.org/10.1002/stem.318. PMID: 20135685; PMCID: PMC2940232.
2. Bucci MK, Bevan A, Roach M III. Advances in radiation therapy: conventional to 3D, to IMRT, to 4D, and beyond. CA Cancer J Clin. 2005;55:117–34.
3. Mallum A, Mkhize T, Akudugu JM, Ngwa W, Vorster M. The role of positron Emission tomog-raphy and Computedn tomographic (PET/CT) imaging for radiation therapy planning: a litera-ture review. Diagnostics. 2023;13:53.
4. Gupta T, Beriwal S. PET/CT-guided radiation therapy planning: from present to the future. Indian J Cancer. 2010;47:126–33.
5. Alongi P, Laudicella R, Desideri I, Chiaravalloti A, Borghetti P, Quartuccio N, Fiore M, Evangelista L, Marino L, Caobelli F, et al. Positron emission tomography with computed tomography imaging (PET/CT) for the radiotherapy planning definition of the biological target volume: part 1. Crit Rev Oncol. 2019;140:74–9.
6. Schinagl DA, Kaanders JH, Oyen WJ. From anatomical to biological target volumes: the role of PET in radiation treatment planning. Cancer Imaging. 2006;6(Spec No A)::S107–16. https://doi.org/10.1102/1470-7330.2006.9017.
7. Daisne JF, Duprez T, Weynand B, Lonneux M, Hamoir M, Reychler H, Grégoire V. Tumor volume in pharyngolaryngeal squamous cell carcinoma: comparison at CT, MR imaging, and FDG PET and validation with surgical specimen. Radiology. 2004;233(1):93–100.
8. Szyszko TA, Cook GJR. PET/CT and PET/MRI in head and neck malignancy. Clin Radiol. 2018;73(1):60–9.
9. Trotter J, Pantel AR, Teo BKK, Escorcia FE, Li T, Pryma DA, Taunk NK. PET/CT imaging in radiation therapy treatment planning: a review of PET imaging tracers and methods to incor-porate PET/CT. Adv Radiat Oncol. 2023;8:101212.
10. IAEA. The role of PET/CT in radiation treatment planning for cancer patient treatment. 2008.
11. Pike LC, Thomas CM, Guerrero-Urbano T, Michaelidou A, Greener T, Miles E, Eaton D, Barrington SF. Guidance on the use of PET for treatment planning in radiotherapy clinical trials. Br J Radiol. 2019;92(1103)
12. EANM. PET/CT radiotherapy planning part 3 a technologist guide. 2012.
13. Wu-Welliver M, Yuh WTC, Fielding JR, Macura KJ, Huang Z, Ayan AS, Backes FJ, Guang J, Moshiri M, Zhang J, Mayr N. Imaging across the life span: innovations in imaging and therapy for gynecologic cancer. Radiographics. 2014;2014(34):1062–81.
14. Bongers ML, Coupe VMH, De Ruysscher D, Lambin P, Oberije C, Uyl-de Groot CA. Pet-based radiotherapy treatment Plannin is highly cost-effective compared to CT-based planning: a model-based evaluation. Value Helath. 2013;16(7):414.
15. Rodriguez J, Mahase S, Roytman M, Pan P, Magge R, Pannullo S, Ivanidze J. Cost-effectiveness of Dotatate PET/MRI for radiation treatment planning in patients with interme-diate-risk meningioma. J Neurol Surg Part B Skull Base. 2021;82(S 02):OD023.

Index